The Home Day-Care Handbook

The Home Day-Care Handbook

A Complete Guide for Establishing Your Own Day-Care Home

By
Sherry Alexander
Portland, Oregon

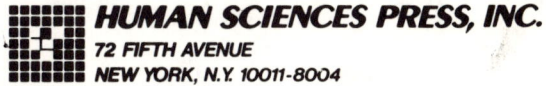

HUMAN SCIENCES PRESS, INC.
72 FIFTH AVENUE
NEW YORK, N.Y. 10011-8004

HV
854
.A67
1987

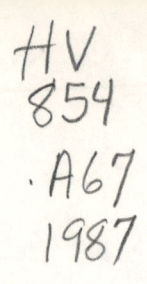

To my husband, Ron, without whose constant encouragement, faith, love, and support, my dream of writing this book would never have been realized.

Copyright © 1987 by Human Sciences Press, Inc.
72 Fifth Avenue, New York, New York 10011
An Insight Book

All rights reserved. No part of this work may be reproduced or utilized in any form or by any means, electronic or mechanical, including photocopying, microfilm and recording, or by any information storage and retrieval system without permission in writing from the publisher.

Printed in the United States of America
987654321

Library of Congress Cataloging-in-Publication Data

Alexander, Sherry.
  The home day-care handbook.

  Includes index.
  1. Family day care—United States—Handbooks, manuals, etc. I. Title.
HV854.A67   1987   362.7′12′0973   86-27184
ISBN 0-89885-344-3 (hard)
     0-89885-365-6 (paper)

CONTENTS

Acknowledgements 9
Preface 11
Introduction 13
1. **RESPONSIBILITIES OF A DAY-CARE PROVIDER** **15**
    To One's Family 18
    To Day-Care Children 20
        Parenting skills 21
        Discipline 22
        Identifying child abuse 24
    To Parents 26
    To Yourself 30
        Handling stress and burnout 31
        Support groups 35
        The realities of day care 37

2. **HOW TO ESTABLISH YOUR BUSINESS** **40**
    Organizing Your Home 40
        Equipment 41
        Cleaning tips 44
    Local Laws 46

Childrens Services Division Rules Governing Standards for Registered Family Day-Care Homes	47
Insurance: Why and How	54
How to Advertise	55
Parent Interviews	57
Agreements, Contracts, and Children's Records	60
The agreement	60
The contract	61
Children's records	61
Scheduling Your Day	63
3. RECORDS TO KEEP FOR TAXES	**65**
IRS Guidelines	66
Use tests	66
Figuring deductions	67
Expenses and Deductions	69
Direct expenses	69
Food expense	71
Indirect expenses	73
Social Security and Self-Employment Tax	74
Establishing an Easy Bookkeeping Procedure	75
4. MEAL PLANNING	**78**
Good Nutrition	78
Good food habits	79
Food problems	79
USDA Guidelines	80
Sample Weekly Menus	83
Food for Fun	85
Breakfast	85
Snacks	91
Lunch/dinner	99
5. TOYS THAT TEACH FUN	**106**
Toys for Each Age	107
Toys to Make	111
Outside Play Areas	115
Toys from tires	121
Other toys	125

6.	**ACTIVITIES, GAMES, CRAFTS, BOOKS**	**128**
	Things to Do Together	129
	Games to Play or Sing	133
	Things to Make	136
	Books to Read	148
7.	**CHILD-SAFE**	**150**
	In the Home	150
	Safety and Sanitary Precautions	155
	Fire Protection	156
	Auto Safety	158
	Poison Prevention	158
	Illnesses	159
8.	**SAMPLE FORMS**	**163**
	Index	194

ACKNOWLEDGEMENTS

I would like to thank my children, Ron, Dawn, Joshua, and April. Thank you for sharing your home and mom with an ever-changing assortment of little children. All of you have given me space to try new ideas. Sure there have been moments of jealousy, but you overcame that feeling with love. I love all four of you very much.

I would also like to thank my mother, Jean. She taught me the value of caring for others. She also helped me to learn the value of living up to my responsibilities and the ability to find joy in the small things in life. Thank you, mom, for being the type of mother that you are.

A special thank-you has to go to Michelle Tennesen of PRO. This is a nonprofit organization that offers support to day-care providers. The Provider's Resource Organization has graciously opened their files to me for research purposes. They have encouraged me when I was down and laughed with me when I was up. Michelle, especially, has been instrumental in the writing of this book. She saw the value where others only saw the improbability.

To the Children's Services Division (CSD) of the state of Oregon goes my gratitude for the wealth of information and business forms they shared with me. I would also like to extend my gratitude to Karen Thomas of Thomas Tax Service for her encouragement and support. It was Karen who saw the value of my work.

Lastly, thank you, Amy and Melody. You have been a pleasure to care for. You are both very special and I shall greatly miss you when you no longer need my care.

PREFACE

"Times have changed!" How often have you heard that phrase? Nowhere will you find more truth in it than in the world of day care. Times have changed, and with them, methods of discipline, of safety, of teaching, and of child rearing. In this era of change, though, there has been very little written to help the day care professional start and maintain a home day-care business.

The Home Day-Care Handbook has been written to aid the home day-care professional in her work. It has evolved from my own experience in the field of home child care.

When I was a child growing up in the 1950s, the need for day care was often filled by neighbors, family, friends, and the teenage babysitter. My mother could only find an ever changing succession of the latter. Every 2 weeks we received a new young sitter, and I stress *young*.

Unfortunately, they were ill-prepared to deal with the four uncontrollable monsters who eagerly greeted them. They must have felt rather like the victims entering the arena in ancient Rome. In all fairness, though, the sitters were not perfect either. They took exquisite delight in the issuing of physical punishment. We retaliated with verbal insults and spy missions, (to get blackmail information). We were children who declined to eat and refused to obey—children even a mother would find it hard to love.

My mother, nevertheless, not only loved us, but was very resourceful. She solved the sitter problem by bestowing the honor on me. Suddenly, I had the responsibility of caring for the children and keeping the house tidy. I learned new ways to keep small children happy out of my own need to survive. I gained extensive experience in the following years caring for relatives', friends', and neighbors' children.

When my husband and I had our first child, I became a working mother. I drew on my experience as a sitter to select one for our son. I soon found that my experience did not keep me from frustration. Sitters often quit without notice. I became accustomed to phone calls at work from sitters who found it hard to deal with temper tantrums, mild colds, or an obstinate child. I worked when I was ill, so as to save my sick days for when our son was ill. All aspects of day care from the provider's side to the parent's side added to my experience.

The last 5 years I have had a registered family day-care home. I have cared for infants and preschoolers as well as our own four children. I have taken classes on the elements of child care, developing parenting skills, child psychology, home management, business management, and living with stress. I have tried to keep abreast of new methods in discipline and in forming relationships. All of this has added to a wealth of experience, and has led to the writing of *The Home Day-Care Handbook*.

INTRODUCTION

This book will provide many helpful hints to the beginning day-care provider who truly wants to be more than just a babysitter. It will also help the established provider by supplying up-to-date information on topics that are related to day care as a business.

Among other things, it offers advice in record-keeping, planning nutritious meals, and menu ideas. Play equipment, toys, games, and crafts are also included.

It also discusses medical emergencies and the need to have parent contracts and agreements. The eighth chapter includes samples of forms to use in your day-care business. These may be copied and used at your discretion.

Day-care providers have long been viewed as inferior to the person who works outside the home. Society has regarded child care as a necessary evil, and this has resulted in the provider developing a low self-esteem.

It is my hope to raise the image of the provider in her own eyes and in the eyes of society. I feel that this can be done effectively when the day-care home is viewed as a business. In order to be respected as such, the day-care home should be organized, in some ways, just as any other business would be.

Day-care providers give much of themselves for most of the day. Stress levels become high when dealing with children and parents. Burnout is a common problem. The turnover rate in day care is astronomical. This only proves that providing day care is not for everyone.

Not every person is equipped with the skills to be a good provider. This book covers the needs of the day-care provider as well as the needs of the children in care. It offers practical suggestions, but not everything will work for everyone. Feel free to pick and choose what information will be of value to you.

Each day-care provider is an individual with special qualities. Often this fact is not recognized. Day-care providers need support from their families, friends, and parents of the children. They give so much, that it is my hope to give them something in return.

Chapter 1

RESPONSIBILITIES OF A DAY-CARE PROVIDER

Are you a day-care provider? Do you open your home and your heart to several small children each day? If so, you are a very special and extremely unique individual. You are one of a growing number of child care providers who have established a home day-care business. Unfortunately, the business you have selected makes many demands. It offers low pay, tremendous stress, little recognition, low self-esteem, and it will leave thousands of tiny fingerprints on everything in your house.

In consideration of the many challenges that you face on a day-to-day basis, you are to be truly commended for selecting such a worthwhile career. You are a child specialist and necessary to our society. Home day-care offers children a place to grow physically, mentally, and emotionally in an environment that is attuned to each child's needs. It is a field that is not open to everyone, regardless of how easy it seems to become a day-care provider. If you want to become a day-care provider, you must thoroughly understand what will be demanded of you. After you are equipped with all the facts, then you must decide if this is the right business for you. If you decide that it is not right, don't feel disheartened. Every profession has demands that can only be met by certain individuals.

"America has truly plunged into the Age of Child Care," according to the June 1985 issue of the *Reader's Digest* (page 103) in the article *Day Care in America* by Carl T. Rowan and David M. Mazie. The authors go on to report that "In 1984, over two-thirds of American women with school-age children worked outside their home." This tremendous increase in working women has caused a vast child care void that is being filled by the services of the home day-care business. It is because of this increased demand that you, as a day-care provider, need to define your responsibilities to your family, to the day-care children, to their parents, and to yourself. If you are to cope successfully with the day-to-day stresses of your chosen career, then you must first list your priorities and values. This has to be done before you take in that first child.

Practically every business, except day care, has a training program. Some states do offer basic training, but often it is inadequate. Lack of training is what causes many day-care providers to burn out within their first year. Child care is not viewed as a rewarding profession. It may rather be viewed as a necessary evil. The day-care provider is often thought of as illiterate and unskilled for any other job. She is looked down on as a limited person whose only function is to watch other people's children without making complaints or gaining recognition. Society in general refuses to acknowledge the great responsibility that the day-care provider has accepted in offering to care for other people's children. It is up to each individual day-care provider to do her best, and thus prove her immense value.

The role of the day-care provider must be filled by a very special person. If you are a day-care provider, then you must realize that the majority of your days will be spent with demanding and often restless children. You will perform tasks that will require a substantial amount of patience, kindness, self-control, resourcefulness, and commitment. You will not have the luxury of retiring to a clean, neat home at the end of a long working day, either. Instead, you will have the privilege of cleaning your own home oftener than would be normal. These are all points to consider before making the decision to become a day-care provider.

Why are these necessary aspects of the business?

Patience is important in almost any business, but it is an essential quality to develop in caring for the needs of children. It is the capacity for calm endurance. Without patience, how could you settle the many disputes that are bound to occur? How could you put up with spilled milk at every meal? How could you allow each child the freedom to grow at his own pace? You will occasionally find it extremely difficult to maintain patience. Children will push you to your limit at various times throughout the day. They do so to test the rules you have established, not to try your patience. But once you have cultivated deep reserves of patience, you will find that you are more at peace with yourself and your day-care children.

Kindness, on the other hand, is demonstrated in everything that you do. Your warmheartedness with children, and a friendly nature, will express your kindness. Your words and actions must demonstrate this trait. With kindness, your day-care children will develop a close relationship with you and you with them. It will also enable you to build self-esteem in every one of the children in your care. Occasionally, you will have to be very tolerant of a particular situation or misbehavior. Kindness on your part will help you to achieve this tolerance.

Each new day will bring with it new tests for your self-control. Melanie may crack Seth in the head at the same time that Michael vomits all over your living room carpet, and baby Jamie falls out of the highchair. Your tension level will undoubtedly rise, but your self-control will prevent you from releasing your anxieties on the children either verbally or physically. There will be days when a padded cell will seem like a dream. Prepare yourself for such days by exercising self-control each day in the *little* things. Then when that inevitable day arrives that Barbara Ann falls into the toilet, and Kelly eats the dogfood, while Jeff and Tami are yanking each other's hair out, you will be ready to exercise self-control. Visualize situations where your attention is needed in three places at once, and how your self-control could stand up to such tests. In a day-care business, crises and uproars are bound to occur. You will probably use the skill of self-control more often than any other skill you develop.

Another valuable quality to develop is resourcefulness. This you can draw upon to devise a new activity, or to solve a difficult problem. Children often need to shift direction during the day. Your resourcefulness will enable the transition to be as smooth as possible. To bring this trait to its full potential you should read any material that will benefit your day-care children. You should also seek help from support groups and from any other source that you find beneficial. By cultivating resourcefulness you will be able to keep little hands, bodies, and minds busy and happy. This is the goal of every day-care provider.

Children will need a commitment from you if they are to build a relationship with you. They need the security of knowing that you will be there for them. It is not easy for children, or for you, to form a bond of trust. It is critical to the well-being of your day-care children that you commit your time, energy, understanding, and even your love to your business. Children will flourish in this type of environment. You, for your own part, will feel a new sense of worth when you realize that you are a day-care provider who does a superior job in a chosen profession.

Exactly what responsibilities you have to everyone concerned must be clear in your mind. You need to completely understand what demands will be placed on you. You must also be aware of your family's rights. All aspects of your home day-care business must be discussed with your family long before that first child arrives. Taking these initial steps will help to assure you of a successful home day-care business.

TO ONE'S FAMILY

Your family will play an important role in your day-care business; so it is essential that they fully understand what will be required of them. The first thing to do is to hold a family meeting with all members present. At this gathering invite your family to explore all the pros and cons of making your home a day-care unit. Follow through on this discussion openly and thoroughly. This will avoid possible conflicts within your family at some later date.

Your family should bring out any questions that come to mind. Will they lose privacy? Will you be too tired to spend quality time with them? When will your daughter get to practice her piano? Will they be expected to help more with the housework? Can they accept the confusion of parents dropping off and picking up their children? Can they share their home peacefully? If your daughter has to put away her doll house for safekeeping, when is she ever going to be able to play with it? Will they be tolerant of small children? How can your son's model plane collection be safeguarded? Do they really understand that some days will be so hectic that you will need both their help and their support? Is your husband willing to have the family dinner served after all the day-care children have gone home?

Your family will also have to face any feelings of jealousy that they may have. This is not an easy feeling to admit to or to deal with. Nevertheless, there will be times when one or more members of your family will feel jealous. Your children may feel that you don't care as much for them after you have day-care children as you did before. At times they may feel they are getting less attention, especially if they get home at the same time a parent arrives. It will be situations like this one that may spark problems with jealousy in your family. Even your spouse is not immune to such feelings. It may sometimes seem to him that you are not giving him the time and undivided interest he expects. Feelings of resentment, jealousy, even outright selfish reactions may arise without warning. Only the negative aspects of child care will register on the family, if you do not thoroughly discuss the ups and downs of carrying on a day-care home before you take that first step into the business.

It is your responsibility to help them see the positive side of having day-care children in your home. Point out, for instance, that young children enjoy older children who take time with them. Young children are very responsive to kindness, and are appreciative to a fault. On the whole, small children are very happy individuals. They will express their happiness with warm hugs, kisses, and smiles. Your family will share the excitement of watching a baby take his first steps, and pronounce his first words. They will have the opportunity of enhancing their own sense of worth by helping the children in your care to learn new things. Even your spouse may at times enjoy helping the children in special projects.

Day care is a business, though, and your family must recognize that fact. As such, most decisions must be made by you. Your family must respect you as the professional that you are. This will be hard for them to adjust to, especially since you will be at home while you conduct your business. Even so, with your help, they can make the adjustment. Always try to keep in mind that you are still a mate to your spouse and a mother to your own children. Do not allow your day-care business to impair your relationship with your family. Take time to reassure them of your love and support. Spend time with them each day. Remember that there is only so much of you to go around. Try not to give everything to your day-care children during the day, so that there is very little of your energy left for your family in the evenings. Return in full measure the love and respect that you expect from your family. Day-care children may come and go, but your own children are the constants in your life.

Day care as a business can easily consume your time, energy—your whole life. You care for children for 10 to 12 hours a day. You cannot leave the office at the end of the day. Since your home is your business, you will often find that it is necessary to arrange your next day's activities, meals, and housekeeping in the evenings. This will require understanding on your family's part. Help them to adjust to the demands of the business you have chosen, spare you the stress of being expected to be Supermom!

TO DAY-CARE CHILDREN

Anyone who cares for young children on a day-to-day basis has accepted an enormous responsibility. As a day-care provider you are expected to nurture and protect the little ones in your care. You need to provide them space to play and to be creative. They need a clean, safe, stimulating environment that will allow them to fulfill their individual growth patterns and to develop into the people that they are to become. Each day will bring new challenges to your parenting skills. You will have to examine your priorities as they relate to each child, because each child will offer different challenges.

You must cultivate a warm relationship with each child. Not

that you are expected to love each child at first sight; but your fondness for children must be evident. Taking pleasure in the personalities of children and their responsiveness to you makes everything easier. As you come to mean a lot to each other, you can absorb some ups and downs.

Children are very sensitive to the attitudes of those close to them. As a home day-care provider, you will become exceptionally close to your day-care children. You will learn to recognize their fears, likes, dislikes, needs, and desires. You will represent an authority figure, but you will also be their friend. These are a few of the aspects of your important role as a day-care provider.

Parenting Skills

Children do the best that they know how, at the time, to meet the task of growing up. If you are to be an effective day-care provider, you must look at *why* a child is behaving the way he is. This is a parenting skill that comes in for much use when dealing with your day-care children. There are many other parenting skills, to be sure; but the first one that you will need to acquire is the ability to identify the developmental task that the child is working on.

Developmental tasks include: learning to control their bodies, getting along with others, communication, independence, problem solving. For instance, when small children ask "What's that?" or "Why?" they are trying to learn the words that are appropriate for use. This will help them in the developmental task of communication. When a three-year-old bites, calls names, threatens or shoves another child, he may be working on the task of independence or cooperation.

As a provider, you can help your day-care children to sometimes find a better way of accomplishing that particular task. This will require a great deal of patience on your part. Sometimes you may run out of options to try. In that case, you must consult with the parent for more ideas. The main goal is to help the child to develop into a caring individual.

Another parenting skill to develop is reflective listening. This will put the child in touch with his own feelings. Children often do not know how to explain their anger, frustration, or even their joy. They do not know the words for what they are feeling. This makes it necessary for you to listen on two levels by paying close attention to children's verbal and nonverbal messages.

In reflective listening you are physically still and paying full attention. This tells the child that you care enough to be quiet and hear him. You can reflect for the child what he is feeling just as a mirror reflects. In this way you can help the child to "see" and clarify the problem bothering him.

A child says, "Amy and Melody didn't want to play with me. There's nothing to do." You must think to yourself what she is feeling like at that moment. Try to think of a feeling word that would describe the emotion you recognize. Then you might say, "It makes it seem like no one cares. You must be feeling left out."

The child may just nod and go off. But you, as the provider, have acknowledged the problem and identified the feeling. You "understand." You don't have to respond to everything a child says with reflective listening. Try, though, to be sensitive to when the child wants to talk or needs your support.

If a child comes to you repeatedly with the same complaint, he may just want your attention. He probably has no intention of solving the problem alone. Simply express your confidence in him by encouraging him to take care of the matter himself. Tell the child that it seems that you cannot help any further. By all means, avoid nagging, criticizing, ridiculing, or lecturing. Treat your day-care children as friends, and practice the golden rule. Allow the children to learn by solving their own problems.

Discipline

Discipline is often thought of as corporal punishment. Actually, it should be viewed as guiding behavior to fit a specific pattern. Day-care providers often encounter children's misbehavior. This sometimes requires an immediate response. One answer would be the use of "time-out."

Time-out is the removal of the child from the activity for a short period of time. For example, one child is continually interrupting as you read a story to your day-care children. You have asked him/her to stop. He/she refuses to, so you remove the child to a quiet place away from the group. You instruct the child that he/she must sit quietly for a certain length of time or you will increase it. When the designated time is over, the child must be brought immediately back to the group. This will reinforce the reason for time-out without your verbally doing so.

Time-out is effective as long as the child is not ridiculed and you are firm in your instructions. Your firmness must be conveyed by your gentle but decided body movements and your tone of voice, which is calm but definite.

Setting reasonable limits is another aspect of discipline. Children need to know what is expected of them. They need to know what the rules are. You must be consistent in setting limits. Children will slowly learn that the limits you have set are to protect them. A reasonable limit would be to not allow climbing on the kitchen table. An unreasonable limit would be to not allow any climbing at all, because it is in children's nature to climb.

You must be consistent, fair, and make no decision without getting all the facts. Show your approval for acceptable behavior. Reinforce acceptable behavior in a positive way. Try to avoid negative words such as "don't," "stop," and "quit." Build confidence in your day-care children. Make them feel that they are important, capable, and worthwhile. Avoid belittling a child. That will only undermine his self-confidence, and in turn make your job more difficult.

Try to examine why a child is misbehaving. Perhaps he/she is defending his/her identity in the day-care unit, or maybe attention is the goal. The child may want power, or may be getting revenge. All of these are possibilities.

If attention is the goal, try to ignore the misbehavior. Pay attention to the child in positive ways when the misbehavior is not occurring.

When gaining power is the objective of the misbehavior, remove yourself from the conflict. Give the child opportunities to use power in constructive ways, by getting him to help you and cooperate.

Revenge is the hardest misbehavior to deal with. Correction often brings out a desire to get even, and the child will only seek more revenge. Thus begins a vicious circle. To help the child overcome misbehavior, stop all criticism entirely. Focus the child's assets and abilities, and above all, don't give up.

Day-care providers should set a good example. They must give praise for good behavior, respect the children and themselves as individuals, and restrict children from behaviors that are harmful to others or destructive to property. Remember, though, that no one is perfect. You will make mistakes; but use these as learning tools when they occur. Using discipline techniques will help, but all of them may not suit your needs. Try positive alternatives to negative discipline. Then you and your day-care children will enjoy your days together.

Identifying child abuse

As a family day-care provider, you need to understand the potential for child abuse. Child abuse and neglect are recognized in every community and are a major national problem. Child abuse has been defined as any condition injurious to the child's physical and emotional health that has been inflicted by parents, guardians, or other care givers. In other words, it is harm inflicted on a child by someone whom the child trusts.

The reasons for child abuse are many and not easy to understand. The most consistent factor is that the abusing parents, guardians, or care givers were often abused themselves as children. As a day-care provider, you are under a moral obligation to report any actual or any suspected cases of child abuse. In some states you are required to do so by law.

What do you look for? There are three major areas holding possible indicators of abuse. The first is the child's behavior. Is it aggressive, disruptive, or destructive? Is the child shy, withdrawn, or passive? Any of these behaviors could be indicators of abuse.

The child's appearance is second. Is physical neglect apparent? Is he repeatedly dressed inadequately for the weather, or not clean? Does the child look undernourished, or always overeat? Is the child always tired?

Parents' attitude is third. When you approach the parents with problems about their child, are they defensive, offended, or "denying"? Do they seem indifferent or unresponsive? Is the relationship with their child, in your observation, lacking in appropriate warmth and spontaneity? Do they show little concern or interest?

Seven major categories of child abuse have been identified. But it must be noted that other factors such as a death, illness, job loss, and planning to move may be highly threatening to the child, resulting in one or more of the possible symptoms of child abuse. The following list was provided by the *Oregon Family Day Care Training Program* pamphlet:

1. Physical Abuse
    a. Bruises on exposed body surfaces.
    b. Child wearing long clothing on a hot day.
    c. Obviously, nonaccidental bruises should be discussed with the child.
    d. If the child seems afraid to go home, he should be questioned.
    e. Cigarette burns.
    f. Broken bones.
2. Nutritional Deprivation
    a. Malnourished because of deliberate underfeeding by parents.
    b. Question children who appear unhealthy, who bring meager lunches, who report no breakfast or being hungry, or who consume huge quantities at school.
    c. If parents are asked, with no response, the following documentation is appropriate:
        1. Document lunch contents for a 2-week period.
        2. Weigh the child on Friday and Monday to document weight loss over the weekend.
        3. Turn the case over the the police or children services.
3. Medical Care Neglect
    a. Child's needs for eye glasses, dental work, or immunizations are not met.
    b. Give parents two reminders, then turn over to authorities.

4. Sexual Abuse
   a. Most cases involve females; about one-half of reported cases are females under 12.
   b. Child most often will not complain because of embarrassment.
   c. Girl is often withdrawn and terrified of any male.
   d. Turn information over to authorities.
5. Emotional Abuse
   a. Difficult to pinpoint.
   b. Child emotionally abused at home will appear emotionally disturbed in classroom.
   c. Referral to family counseling or mental health clinic.
   d. If parents refuse, you can report to children's services.
6. Severe Hygiene Neglect
   a. Child smells of urine and is teased by other children.
   b. Encourage parents to improve hygiene.
   c. If parent refuses, turn over to authorities.
7. Educational Neglect
   a. Oregon laws provide for guaranteed school attendance.

In all 50 states, the reporting person is protected against any type of liability suit. If you suspect child abuse, it is your responsibility to report it. In some states you are required by law to do so. Failure to comply with the law can result in prosecution. Take time to learn your state's laws regarding the reporting of child abuse. In such instances, intervention is critical.

Above all, remember who you are. As a day-care provider you have definite responsibilities to your day-care children. Recognize those responsibilities and you will indeed be a quality provider, a very special person. You also have definite responsibilities to your day-care parents. Exactly what these entail is discussed next.

TO PARENTS

When children are left in your care, parents are often worried. They wonder if Patti will make friends, will Matthew be changed often enough so his diaper rash won't get worse, will the provider be able to understand what Toby tries to tell her, and if shy Jessica will get enough attention. Sometimes their feelings of guilt over leaving their child may cause them to overreact to their children and you. They may become argumentive, demanding, picky, or even jealous if you are well liked by the child. Parents may even feel that you are replacing them in their role with their child.

It is important for you to understand the parent's point of view in relation to you as the provider. You need to understand their doubts and anxiety over leaving their child. You need to have an open line of communication between yourself and the parents, and to develop a good relationship with them.

Communication is the key to developing that good relationship. How do you go about establishing good communication with your day-care parents? How do you let them know that you are there to work with them and to support them as parents? Here are some ideas:

1. Tell the parents that they are the important people in their child's life. Don't be a parent to your day-care children. You are there to provide care in the parent's absence.
2. Reassure the parents by listening to them. Take their ideas and values seriously. Try to reenforce these ideas and values in their children.
3. Respect their right to privacy and confidentiality. If their child is sharing private information from home, change the subject of the talk.
4. Let parents know that you are available for them too. Let them know that you will make time for them if they want to talk.
5. Keep parents posted on what you are doing with their children. Let them know in advance about field trips and special events. Encourage the children to take home art work. Share any educational projects you are working on with the parents. Remember that parents enjoy hearing about their child's day. Try to let them know, briefly, what went on while their child was in your care.
6. Let the parents know you. Share some of your ideas and values with the parents. Let them know you are a complete person just as they are.

All of these approaches will help to develop an open, honest, and positive relationship. As a provider, though, you will also need to establish rules, to minimize understandings. Some reasonable rules are:

1. You have a starting time and a quitting time, just as they do.
2. You need to be paid on time. You have bills to pay and day care is your business.
3. If there are times when a parent is late in picking up their child, you have a late fee that must be paid when their child is picked up.
4. Even though it seems out of the question to expose well children to one who is symptomatic, many providers do care for ill children. There are basically two reasons for this; parents' loss of income and provider loss of income. If you decide to take care of children who are ill, what does that include? For example, will you take them when they have colds, allergies, diarrhea, fevers, sore throats, or chicken pox? Make sure all parents are aware of your decision. In some states, a registered or licensed provider must not care for ill children. Check your state's regulations.
5. You have a family and a life outside of your business; you need time to rest. You do not want phone calls after business hours unless it is in regard to the child's arrival the next day.
6. You expect parents to come to the door to pick up and drop off their child.
7. You expect parents to make sure their children are clean and in clean clothing on their arrival.
8. You will inform parents of any procedures that both you and they need to follow for the safety and security of their children.
9. Ask parents to set up appointments with you to discuss any problem area. If they just drop in, you may have another appointment.

These are only a few of the rules that might apply to your day-care business. Each provider will have her own set of rules that are important to her. The essential thing is to let the parents know what your rules are.

Occasionally, problems will arise in spite of an open relationship. What then? How do you express your feelings and needs without closing the door to further communication? This is not an easy task. You must be positive and employ tact. Speak clearly, and in a sufficiently direct way that parents understand correctly what you are trying to get across. Choose words that are as accurate and specific in their meaning as possible. Don't make your listener have to second-guess you. Think about what you are going to say before you say it. Check your tone of voice and body language to make sure they match your words.

Be honest in what you say. If you are not honest, then your body language may give you away. For instance, if you say "I think you are doing fine as a parent," but your tone of voice is questioning, or if your nervous fidgeting suggests you wish you were someplace else, the parent will pick up on these signals and become confused: ("What is she driving at?"). This in turn may cause the parent to become agitated and angry. ("She's not playing with a full deck!")

When approaching the discussion of a problem, do it in a positive way. Talk about your feelings and needs. Avoid blaming or accusing the parent or the child. Give what is called an "*I* message." This expresses your feelings, and states why you feel the way you do. This is not being egotistical; it is being real.

Suppose you have a parent who has fallen into the habit of paying you late. You could approach the parent and say "*You* get paid on a regular basis, and I want to be paid on a regular basis. Either pay me on time, or find someone else to take care of your child." How would the parent react to such an ultimatum? To save face, she would almost have to accept the challenge and say, "Fine, I'll make other arrangements!"

What if you used an "*I* message" instead? Suppose you said, "I've been feeling really frustrated lately. I have bills that need to be paid on time, and it is very hard for me to do that when I am paid late." In this statement you are talking about yourself and your own needs, which are your first concern, and properly so. You are not accusing anyone. Rather, you are letting the parent know that you have a problem, and are allowing the parent to take some initiative in solving it.

You must also listen carefully and thoughtfully to what the

parent says. Give parents your undivided attention. Don't interrupt. Let them know that what they have to say is important to you. Sometimes people have difficulty expressing themselves clearly. They may say what they don't really mean. It is up to you to sort out the information the parent is giving to determine what is really being said. Try to distinguish whether the parent is worried, angry, perplexed, defensive, frustrated, or what. Watch the parent's body language. Is she relaxed, or is she obviously tense?

All of this will help you to determine what the parent is really saying; but you could be wrong. So do a little more checking. Ask the parent if you are interpreting her correctly. If you are wrong, the parent will correct you. If you are right, the parent will confirm it. Either way, there is a "meeting of minds," and usually, increased cordiality.

This process of giving and receiving clear and precise information will help you to eventually come to an understanding. Once the problem is defined, you can find a solution together.

Maintaining open lines of communication will help you to develop a good relationship with your day-care parents. Recognizing your responsibilities to them will make your job a lot easier. But what about you? Do your feelings really count? How can you prevent burnout? All of these questions are answered next, as your responsibilities to yourself are defined.

TO YOURSELF

It is 6 o'clock in the evening and the sun is setting over your neighbor's house. Little Tommy is waving goodbye from the front seat of his mother's car. He was the last of your five day-care children to leave. As you close the door, you glance around the room that is strewn with toys. You even make a feeble attempt to pick up a doll as you sink into a nearby chair.

This has been an especially hectic and long day. A few minutes of peace and quiet would be welcome. Your mind begins to wander. What did Susan's mother mean when she said that Susan sure looked tired? Why did Jeremy spread peanut butter all over the piano? Did Jessie and Kimberley have to fight all day?

How did the toilet get plugged for that third time? Just at the moment that you are mentally letting go of a stressful day, you hear, loud and clear, "Mom, are we going to have dinner? I'm starved!" Your moment of peace and quiet has been shattered. You have been jerked back into the ongoing world of homelife. You must face the fact that your day is not over. Slowly you give up the comfort of your chair, and begin putting toys away. Before long, dinner has been served, and you are once again clearing the table while your family pursues their interests. You stave off exhaustion in order to spend some time with your spouse and children.

Before you know it—bedtime arrives. After a hot shower to relax, you literally crawl into your bed. You can still feel the bruise on your thigh from the kick that Jessie gave you when you put her in time-out for fighting with Mary. But, the weekend is only 4 days away. Your eyes close for what seems only moments, when the alarm clock goes off.

Slowly you get out of your warm, comfortable bed. You hurry to get dressed and beat your children to the bathroom. Soon you are standing, smile in place, at the front door. In rapid succession you warmly greet Jessie, Mary, Jeremy, Suzie, and little Tommy. Another day has begun, and now it's only 3 days until the weekend!

Does this sound familiar to you? As a home day-care provider, your day-to-day responsibilities are great. You are expected to provide loving care for the children whom you take into your home. You are to provide protection from hazards, as well as with learning activities to stimulate them mentally and physically. This job has many rewarding aspects, but like most complex jobs, it presents problems, too.

The major problem that you, as a day-care provider, will face is stress. What type of stress will you be faced with? How is stress related to provider burnout? How can stress be met?

Handling stress and burnout

Stress results when you are subjected to pressure, strain, or confusion. Every day you, as the provider, are faced with the stress of soothing sometimes sad or angry children. You have to meet too many demands on your energies. There is also the stress of everyday living, and the stress of working with parents. The many responsibilities you have pile up the pressure. Finally, there is the type of stress that is unique to day-care providers. That stress is related to using your home to operate your day-care business. It is this type of stress that can cause the most problems for a day-care provider.

You have willingly opened your home to small children, true, but that does not ease the feelings of isolation, low self-esteem, or frustration. A person's home is usually an oasis, a refuge from the world. It is a place where stress can usually be minimized, and is often viewed as a kind of sanctuary. But, in a day-care home your oasis becomes a hub of activity. It is constantly used and abused. You are forever cleaning up after children.

You become isolated from your peers. Your day revolves around the care and feeding of small children. You have to speak their language. Their demands cause you to continually give out more than you receive back. Soon, without support, you become a victim of low self-esteem.

You begin to lose sight of the rewards of your job, and dwell on the negative aspects. You may feel resentful towards the children in your care because of the daily demands on your time. Or you may withdraw from friends and family. Frustration and apathy often develop next, and before you realize it, you are completely burned out. You have no resources left to give. You are like a kerosene lamp that has been allowed to burn dry. How can this be prevented before it happens? How can you avoid provider burnout?

Here are four possible ways:

1. Be aware of some common stressful situations and preferred ways of meeting them.
2. Be aware of the signs of stress and ways to relieve them.
3. Determine what kinds of behavior are acceptable to you and take steps to prevent unacceptable behavior.
4. Be aware of community resources to be used for field trips with the children and to support you.

1. *Common stress.* You as a day-care provider are aware of many possible stressful situations. You not only have to handle confrontations, but you also must face day-to-day problems. Many of the problems you meet on a daily basis can be controlled. This will reduce stress. How *do* you avoid daily problems? The best way is to organize the day-care environment. When you systematize your home and your daily routine, you alleviate much of the day-to-day stress. For instance, if everything is in its place, you will be much calmer than if you are constantly tripping over toys. True, these are small irritations, but they can build toward a major crisis (refer to Chapter 2 for ways to organize your home).

The daily or weekly routine, when organized, will lessen possible stressful situations. Children, on the whole, have a very strong sense of order. They need the security of knowing what will happen next. Try to plan meals, snacks, naps, and playtimes at the same time each day. The children will be much calmer and you will have less stress.

Another factor to consider is the noise level of your home. The louder the noise, the higher the stress level. To keep this level within normal limits try using a quiet voice when you are speaking. You will also need to talk with the children about the concepts of loud and soft. This is especially important with small children. Often they do not understand the difference between words such as loud and soft.

Plan quiet activities that do not increase the noise level. For example, use a carpeted area to play with blocks. Remember, though, to plan noisy activities too. Children need to have time to be loud and expressive. It is vital to their well-being that they be allowed this outlet. Outside play is the ideal activity for this. When children are able to run and shout, under supervision, it is easier for them to be quiet later in the day.

2. *Signs of stress and ways to relieve it.* Everyone needs stress to motivate them to achieve their goals. You, however, as a day-care provider, often undergo unhealthy stress. This is the type that causes stomach and nervous problems, and family discord. Stress like this arises not only from the noise and confusion, but also from the demands made of you. You must recognize the signs of stress so that you can relieve it.

Probably the most obvious sign of stress is tension. This can be recognized in tight shoulder muscles, clenched fists, grinding of teeth, and even in headaches. For example, suppose that Jeff drops his plate on the floor. You become slightly irritated, but it was an accident, so you bend down and begin picking up the plate. As you are on the floor, Mark spills his milk on your head. Now your shoulders begin to get tight. Later in the day, Jennifer breaks your living room window. Now you are gritting your teeth and clenching your hands. Your head begins to ache. Your tension is reaching a stress crisis. How can you relieve it?

One way is to take a few deep breaths. As you do, contract and relax your muscles. If you can lie down a few minutes in absolute silence after the children leave, this will help too. Try massaging your head at the temple areas. Apply a cold compress to your eyes. Any one or all of these ideas may prove beneficial to relieving tension caused by stress. At the end of your day, take a long hot bath or go for a quiet walk. If you have excess energy to burn, try walking vigorously. Talking to an understanding friend or spouse can also do wonders to relieve stress.

Other signs of stress may include anger, frustration, loss of or increase in appetite, nervousness and insomnia. To find alternate methods of coping with stress, enroll in a stress workshop. Often local colleges make these available for a small fee. You could also contact your area's Department of Mental Health for information. The local library is another valuable resource. You will find many books on stress on your library's shelves.

3. **Acceptable and unacceptable behavior.** Before you decide to become a day-care provider, you must determine what behaviors you are willing to accept. This will be a determining factor in selecting the ages of the children you will offer to care for. For example, if drooling and crying are behaviors that you cannot accept, then you should not take care of infants. All infants will drool when teething and will cry when their needs are not met, and sometimes when you don't know why. This is normal behavior for this age group. You can avoid increased stress by recognizing behaviors that are common in children.

There are behaviors, though, that can be changed or avoided if you find them unacceptable. Once you have established what they are you can set up guidelines to be followed by the children. For instance, if you cannot tolerate roughhousing, set guidelines regarding it that are easily understood. Explain that running, jumping, and wrestling need to be done in a designated place so that no one will be hurt, nor damage done.

You must always offer positive alternatives to undesirable behavior. If you find that a child is repeatedly allowing her nose to run, explain and demonstrate the proper way to wipe the nose. You can even supply the child with her own box of Kleenex. Soon the undesirable behavior will disappear, and you will have less stress to deal with.

4. Community resources. Every community has its own valuable resources to be tapped. There are many that offer places of interest for children. Field trips to these places will help both you and the children counter day-to-day stress by offering a break in the routine.

Perhaps you could plan a field trip once a month, or even once a week. The children will eagerly look forward to these. Try visiting a bakery, a fire station, a school, the zoo, a fast-food restaurant, the police station, or a produce market. The possibilities are endless. You could even ask the children for ideas. A change in scenery for a few hours will help a lot.

There are many resources available for you as the provider, too, such as support groups and outside activities.

If your community offers evening concerts, attend them. Take a picnic supper with you and enjoy the relaxed atmosphere. Basically, you need to take advantage of any resource that will help you to unwind. This will restore your energies to meet the demands put upon you by your day-care business.

Support groups

You are not alone! You are unique, yes, and so are your problems, but you as a day-care provider are not alone. There are others just like you. Together, you can conquer many of the obstacles that arise in caring for other people's children. That is why support groups are so important.

Only another provider will understand the stress that is

generated on a daily basis by a business with no days off, no sick days, and with limited financial returns. Only another provider will understand the feelings of boredom and isolation. Since this is in fact the only way to be understood, talk to another provider. Join or create a support network of day-care providers. This may not be easy to accomplish at first, but keep trying. It will not only bring lasting benefits to you, but also to other providers in your area.

In Oregon such a group was established, called the Provider's Resource Organization, or PRO. As of February 1985 PRO was approved by the State of Oregon as a nonprofit organization. PRO's philosophy and statement of purpose are as follows:

PRO philosophy. The Provider's Resource Organization or PRO was founded by day-care providers who recognized the high-stress nature of day care and felt a support network should be in place.

PRO was founded for all providers regardless of state registration, USDA affiliation, sex, race, or religion. Its only requirement for membership is that day care be run in a manner that does not jeopardize the health and well-being of the children. All providers are viewed with love, compassion, and understanding.

The organization does not dictate how a day-care business should be run. It does not advocate one style of discipline or teaching over another but rather encourages what works best with each provider's family, talents, and resources. It will offer suggestions, information, and ideas as requested.

PRO encourages cooperation with other agencies interested in child care and upgrading the stature of child care. This benefits all—child, provider, and parent. Be a PRO.

PRO's statement of purpose. To recognize child care as an honest and legitimate profession.

To upgrade the profession in the manner by which the providers run their business and the quality of child care they provide.

To elevate the status of care givers in the eyes of the provider, the public, and the private sector.

To enhance provider life through support, training, and burnout recognition.

To extend love, compassion, and consideration to all providers regardless of sex, race, or creed.

The realities of day care

A day-care provider always hopes that each day will pass in relative peace and harmony. However, each day that you care for children will bring some unforeseen problems. This is to be expected when you open your home to children of various ages and stages of development.

The day-to-day care of children can be both rewarding and frustrating. It can be fun or it can be tiring and discouraging. Usually, it is some of both. By being aware of the realities of day care, you can prepare yourself to handle most situations that result from children's behavior. Following is a list of special problems that you must be able to deal with. Try to understand why the child is reacting in the way he is. Could he be angry, tired, upset, frustrated, or hurt? Then consider what methods you will use in each situation. Will you remove the child to another area, give time out, change the activity, or ignore the problem at that moment? Remember to choose methods that will encourage the child to develop self-control. Most of all, find ways to develop self-control on your own part. Never yell at, embarrass, shame, or threaten a child. Remain calm. Talk with him. Harsh punishment usually makes a child withdraw into himself. He becomes resentful or may doubt his ability to do what is required of him. Try to think instead of react. Some common problems are:

1. Biting
2. Lying
3. Destructiveness
4. Throwing
5. Refusal to share
6. Temper tantrums
7. Hitting
8. Stealing
9. Hyperactivity

10. Jealousy
11. Sleep problems
12. Screaming and yelling
13. Demanding attention
14. Anxiety or frustration
15. Phobias
16. Lack of respect for people or property
17. Hurting others
18. Quarreling or arguing
19. Balkiness
20. Aggressiveness
21. Lack of cooperation

There are other realities of day care that you must be aware of that are not behavior issues. Most are directly related to the children's parents. A few are:

1. Lack of cleanliness
2. Head lice or scabies
3. Improper clothing for the weather
4. Bad manners
5. Late arrival or pickup of child
6. Late payment or nonpayment of fees
7. Improper dental hygiene
8. Lack of medical care
9. Parental jealousy
10. Parental guilt
11. Low parental self-esteem
12. Parental demands and advice
13. Phone calls from parents after day-care hours

The problems and situations that have been mentioned are only a few. There are many more. Some will occur several times a day. Some may never happen. Then there are those that happen two or three at a time. Remember to multiply the likely events of day care by the number of children in your care. This will help you prepare for the realities and develop skill and confidence in managing them.

You can make a difference in a small child's life—if you are dedicated, loving, and prepared. To do so is to succeed in your chosen profession. For, after all, you are a businesswoman. And, as such, you are a unique individual.

Chapter 2

HOW TO ESTABLISH YOUR BUSINESS

Now that you are fully aware of the responsibilities of a day-care provider, you are ready to establish your business. The prerequisite for any successful business is organization. This is especially true for home day care. Since you must take into account the needs and desires of your own family, complete organization may take extra time. Don't allow yourself to become frustrated. You can do it.

Most families do not want the home day-care business to interfere with their home life. Certain rooms in the home may have to be placed off-limits to the children in your care, in order to maintain peace within the family unit. This may also apply to certain items in the home that your own children do not wish to share. It is important to consider all areas pertaining to your family when organizing the home for day care.

ORGANIZING YOUR HOME

The first step requires listing all areas and items to be considered off-limits. This list should be used as your basic floor

HOW TO ESTABLISH YOUR BUSINESS   41

plan. Next, review the following questionnaire to determine what your assets and needs are:

1. Where will my active area be?
2. Where will the children sit to put puzzles together and color?
3. Where are the children going to sleep?
4. Is my home equipped for feeding young children?
5. What type of outdoor play area does my home offer?
6. What changes do I need to make in my home to save time and energy in its maintenance?
7. Where will I put ill children?
8. Do I have a place to store toys, games, and materials?
9. How many children will I care for?
10. What ages do I have to prepare for?
11. Is my home prepared for the toileting needs of young children?
12. Where will I keep my records and files on the children?
13. How can I make my home safe for young children? (stairs, windows, etc.)

Taking time to calculate your needs, to begin your business properly, will reduce stress later. Each day-care home will have different requirements. That is to be expected because each day-care provider is different. This is why it is so important for you to prepare in advance.

Equipment

When you decide to become a day-care provider, you suddenly become faced with providing equipment for a small army. Where do you start?

Basically, you will need sleeping, eating, and playing equipment. The types will vary with the ages of children in your care. For instance, an infant will need a crib to sleep in, whereas a four-year-old can use a bed or a mat. Since most day-care providers take three to five children of varying ages, the equipment needs can be considerable. But try to keep it simple. After all, parents often find it a financial burden to prepare for only one infant. You may have to prepare for two.

To help you decide what equipment is necessary, here are some guidelines.

Infant to one year will require:

> a crib or portacrib or playpen
> mattress
> bumper pad
> sheets, blankets, lap pads
> high chair
> infant seat (optional)
> infant swing (optional)
> infant walker (optional)
> car seat
> stroller or backpack
> disposable diapers
> toys
> mobiles
> storage for diaper bag from home

1 year to 18 months will require:

> crib or playpen (portacrib is too small)
> mattress
> bumper pad
> sheets, blankets, lap pads
> high chair
> car seat
> stroller
> disposable diapers
> nonspill cup
> potty chair
> toys and books
> storage for diaper bags from home

18 months to 2½ years will require:

>   playpen (optional)
>   sleeping mat
>   slumber bag or blanket
>   high chair
>   car seat
>   stroller
>   disposable diapers
>   potty chair
>   toys and books
>   storage for things from home

2 ½ years to 3 years will require:

>   sleeping mat
>   slumber bag or blanket
>   car seat
>   potty chair
>   toys and books
>   cups and utensils easy to grasp

3 years to 4 years will require:

>   sleeping mat
>   slumber bag or blanket
>   car seat
>   toys and books

4 years and up will require:

>   sleeping mat
>   slumber bag or blanket
>   toys, books, etc.

Cleaning tips

Having your own day-care business takes a lot of elbow grease. Children can be messy and this makes cleaning an ongoing task. To maintain order, you will need to accomplish certain tasks on a regular basis. Some will have to be done daily, others weekly.

It is important to maintain health and safety standards in your home. Refer to Chapter 7 on Child-Safe for guidelines.

Your daily cleaning before the children arrive should not take any longer than 30 minutes. Here is a suggested list of eight tasks, to which you may wish to add, as your home setting requires.

1. Sweep or vacuum all floors.
2. Disinfect toilet and clean sink.
3. Wash any dirty dishes.
4. Damp-mop eating area and bathroom.
5. Empty wastebaskets.
6. Make sure medicine cabinets and cleaning supply cupboards are locked.
7. Check each room to make sure that cleaning agents, medicines, cigarettes, etc. are put away.
8. Make sure all areas that are off-limits are closed off.

Throughout the day messes will happen. Try to take care of them quickly. After eating, clear and wash dishes right away. Take high chair trays directly to the sink to clean. This will eliminate dried food collecting on the underside of the tray. Put a sheet of plastic or newspapers under high chairs to save time in cleaning your floors. When children are small, use bottom-heavy cups for drinking. This will cut down on the spilled milk.

Teach your day-care children to put away toys after they are finished playing with them. This will help lessen the clutter that occurs when several children are in your care. The same applies to craft projects. When they are completed, help the children clean up both the space used and themselves.

An effective cleaning schedule is vital to your day-care home. You have to take steps to sanitize it in order to reduce the risk of illness to your family and your day care children. This is why it is necessary to also have a weekly cleaning schedule. Here are eight basic guidelines:

1. Wash all bedding and clothes used by the children.
2. Wash toys. Put washable toys in nylon bags and wash in the bathtub. Be sure to add a germicide to the water. Rinse well and hang to dry. Wipe down other toys and play equipment.
3. Clean out all toy boxes. Check for broken toys. Reassemble games.
4. Wipe off all finger- and handprints on woodwork and windows. Dust all furniture.
5. Thoroughly vacuum, sweep, and mop all floors.
6. Clean kitchen thoroughly. Wash down cabinets, counters, appliances, table, and chairs. Mop floor. Clean refrigerator.
7. Disinfect toilet, sink, and tub. Disinfect floor area surrounding toilet.
8. Plan menu and activities for the week. Shop accordingly.

Experiment with cleaning schedules to determine which is best for you. You may want to add to or delete some steps from the basic guidelines. You will find that after experimenting with various cleaning schedules, the one that you select will require minimal time to complete. Each task will be accomplished quickly when you are prepared.

Since your day-care business is conducted in your family home, you may find that some cleaning chores are endless. This is a contributing factor to provider burnout. It can seem impossible to accomplish everything that needs to be done. Your days will seem to begin and end with cleaning. You may feel that you are doing this from dawn until after the last member of your family is in bed.

How can you survive such demands? You can delegate some responsibilities to your family. Ask for their help in cleaning and in meal preparation. Teach your children how to prepare their own breakfasts. This may allow you a few minutes to relax (like, look at the morning paper) before the day-care children arrive.

Make a list of several household chores. Ask your children and spouse to divide these among themselves everyday. This can be accomplished by writing each task on a separate 3 × 5 card. Each family member will choose a personal task (making their bed) and a family task (take out garbage or clean bathroom sink) to accomplish daily. Family members could rotate the tasks on a daily or weekly basis. This would allow everyone a change of pace.

Hold a family meeting to determine which task each family member prefers. Stress the importance of working together as a team. Ask all family members to write down activities, appointments, and meetings on a central calendar. This will help in planning your schedule.

When doing laundry, wash only those clothes that are placed in the hamper. Explain to your family in advance that you do not have time to search for dirty clothing. After folding laundry, put each family member's clothing in a separate basket or box. Have each person put their own clothing away. Do the same with any clothes that require ironing, unless a member of your family volunteers to do that task.

At the end of the week, try to get your weekly cleaning quickly out of the way. Maybe you and your family could work together to accomplish this on Friday evenings. Then, Saturdays and Sundays would be basically chore-free. Everyone needs a time with minimal demands. When you schedule your cleaning needs properly, you will find that keeping your home clean requires a lot of effort—but very little time.

LOCAL LAWS

Before establishing your day-care business, you must check what the local laws are and what they entail. Each state has its own requirements. Contact your state's children's services department to find out what governmental branch handles day care. Then, carefully and diligently find out exactly what procedure you must follow to establish your business. You will find that in some states, the laws are so restrictive that compliance would be too costly. If this is the case, remember that being a professional does not rest on a license or certificate of registration, but on supplying the best care possible.

In order to illustrate the important of such rules, *The Rules Governing Standards for Registered Family Day-Care Homes* from the state of Oregon have been included here. This is only for your general information, and does not eliminate the necessity for you to check on local laws. Verifying rules, regulations, standards, and laws are a fundamental business practice. You are a professional, and as such need to live up to the laws of the day-care business. Meeting official standards, whether they apply only to registered or licensed providers, demonstrates the quality of professionalism that you have attained. All children deserve a clean, safe environment that will allow them to develop to their full potential. This can be accomplished if you comply with your state's guidelines.

CHILDREN'S SERVICES DIVISION RULES GOVERNING STANDARDS FOR REGISTERED FAMILY DAY-CARE HOMES

412–10–400 Applicability and Purpose of Rules

1. These rules set forth Children's Services Division (CSD) standards to be used for reviewing and, if appropriate, registering family day-care homes serving one or more children whose care is purchased by Children's Services Division, or by any other agency which requires its clients to use facilities that must meet applicable state and/or federal requirements. These rules also apply to any person who voluntarily applies to be registered.
2. Those child day-care providers who were issued a certificate of compliance by CSD prior to September 30, 1981 shall be required to meet the registration standards in Rules 412–10–400 through 412–10–435 as amended effective 10/1/81. Certified providers will be considered registered through the date of expiration of their certificate.

412–10–405 Definitions

1. "Care Giver" means any person, including the provider, who cares for the children in the registered family day-care home and works directly with the children.

48   THE HOME DAY-CARE HANDBOOK

2. "Child" means a child under 15 years of age.
3. "Day Care" means care provided to a child during a part of the 24 hours of one day, with or without compensation.
4. "Day-Care Child" is any child, related to the provider or not, who does not reside in the home and for whom the provider has supervisory responsibility in the temporary absence of the parent.
5. "Division" and "CSD" means the Children's Services Division, or the Administrator, or staff of the Division.
6. "Parent" means parent(s), custodian(s) or guardian(s) currently exercising physical care and custody of the children.
7. "Provider" means the person in the registered family day care home who is responsible for the children in care and in whose name the registration is made.
8. "Registered Family Day-Care Home" means any home which has applied for registration under these rules and which has been notified of their registration by CSD.

412-10-410 Certificate of Registration

1. The applicant must apply for registration on the form supplied by CSD.
2. Registration is in effect only after the applicant has been so notified by CSD.
3. The registration is valid for a maximum of 2 years. It is not transferable to another location or individual. Reapplication is required for a new address.
4. The applicant will complete the self-evaluation form. Visits by agency staff will be made on a sample basis.
5. These rules apply only during the hours children are in care.

412-10-415 Children in Care

1. Number and Ages of Children—There shall be no more than five day-care children in care at any one time. No more than two children, including the provider's own children, shall be under two years of age. Children related to the provider but who reside elsewhere may be day-care children. See Definitions "Day-Care Child."

2. The following records must be kept by the registered provider:
   a. Daily attendance record.
   b. Information and Authorization Form for each child.
   c. Emergency Medical Treatment Form accepted by local medical facility for each child.
   d. Medication administered.
   e. Accidents, injuries, and communicable diseases.
3. Taking Children for Care—at the time a child enters care, the care giver must give parents a copy of "Registered Family Day Care: Parents and Providers Working Together."

412–10–410 The Day Care Giver and Family

1. Age, Health and Character
   a. Age and Health—The care giver must be at least 18 years old and in such physical and mental health as will not adversely affect the child in care.
   b. No one can be in the registered home who has been convicted of a crime of immoral conduct or convicted of violating a criminal statute that protects children, or who has demonstrated behavior which may have a detrimental affect on a child.
   c. If additional information is needed to assess an applicant's ability to care for children, references on an evaluation by a physician, psychiatrist, or other qualified person may be required by CSD.
2. There should be no other employment during the hours children are in care. The provider or a substitute care giver who is at least 18 years old must be on the premises during all the hours children are in care.
3. Foster care may be combined with day care only with the permission of the foster care certification worker.
4. The home must be the residence of the applicant. There may be one applicant per household.
5. Any registered day-care provider, who has reasonable cause to believe that a child in care has suffered abuse (physical injury, neglect which leads to physical harm, or sexual molestation) must report the incident to CSD or to a law enforcement agency.

412-10-425 The Home

1. Safety
    a. Indoor space shall allow a minimum of 35 square feet per child exclusive of bathrooms and hallways.
    b. Outdoor play area shall be free from hazards and be protected by fencing or some type of barrier if it is accessible to a street, drainage ditch, or any other hazard. In homes serving children under five years of age with an unfenced play area, the provider shall accompany the children outdoors.
    c. All floor levels and rooms used by the children for play and napping shall have two usable exits.
    d. All exposed electrical receptacles in rooms used by children under age five shall have hard-to-remove protective caps.
    e. Clear glass panels in sliding doors and storm doors shall be clearly marked.
    f. Protection shall be provided from fireplaces, space heaters, wood stoves, stairways, and all other hazardous conditions.
    g. An emergency light source, such as a flashlight, shall be readily available and in operating condition.
    h. Items of potential danger (medicine, drugs, cleaning supplies and equipment, paints, plastic bags, aerosols, detergents, etc.) shall be kept under lock and away from food service supplies (locks may include hook latches).
    i. Firearms, ammunition, and other potentially hazardous equipment shall be kept under lock. Guns shall be disassembled, when possible. Ammunition shall be stored separately from firearms.
    j. Hot water heaters shall be equipped with a safety release valve.
    k. There must be a telephone in operating condition. Emergency telephone numbers for fire department, ambulance, and police must be on the telephone.
    l. There must be a container of first aid supplies available for use and out of the reach of children. It shall contain bandages, gauze pads, a wound cleaning agent (such as

soap or sealed moisture towelettes), scissors, and tweezers. First aid supplies must be taken on field trips.
2. Health
   a. Unless all children in care are from one family, ill children shall not be accepted for day care.
   b. An ill child must be isolated from other children until picked up by the parent.
   c. Room temperature of at least 68 degrees Fahrenheit shall be maintained while children are awake.
   d. The building and grounds, toys, equipment, and furniture shall be maintained in a clean, sanitary, and hazard-free condition.
   e. Drinking water shall meet Health Division standards.
   f. Dogs shall have rabies vaccinations as recommended by animal control agencies.
   g. An individual bed or crib with individual bedding appropriate to the season shall be provided for each child. Family beds may be used. If the parents so request, siblings may share the same bed.
3. Nutrition
   a. Lunch and morning and afternoon snacks shall be given by the provider. When attendance is prior to 7 a.m. a child shall be offered a breakfast if it was not provided by the parent(s). When the planned attendance is after 6:30 p.m. a child shall be offered dinner if it will not be provided by the parent(s).
   b. All meals shall include at least one serving from the Basic Four food groups (bread and cereal; fruits and vegetables; milk and milk products; meat, fish, poultry, and vegetable protein foods, such as legumes, i.e., dried beans and peanut butter). All snacks shall be selected from the Basic Four Food Groups.
   c. There shall be no more than 3½ hours between meals and snacks.
   d. Grade A pasteurized and fortified milk shall be served to children. Powdered milk may be used only for cooking. The serving of raw milk is prohibited. No low fat or skimmed milk shall be served to a child under two years of age without written parental consent.

e. Home frozen or commercially canned jam, jelly, fruit and vegetables may be served. All meat, fish, and poultry served must be USDA inspected.
f. Honey shall not be served to children under 12 months of age.

412–10–430 The Care Given to Children

1. Children must be supervised at all times. The provider must give the children's needs first priority, assuring that they get adequate care and attention. This will often mean taking fewer than five children.
2. If a child becomes ill, he or she must be separated from the other children and the parents notified immediately. If the illness is serious, the physician named on the emergency medical treatment form must be notified or the child must be taken to the hospital or clinic named on the form.
3. The provider may administer medication to a child under the following conditions:
   a. For prescription medications, there must be written authorization from the parent to administer the medication, and it must be administered in accordance with a physician's current orders.
   b. For nonprescription medications, the parents' written instructions must include the name of the medication, circumstances under which it should be administered, dosage, and frequency of administration.
   c. There shall be a written record maintained of medications administered listing, as a minimum, the name of the child, the name of the person administering the medication, date, time, dosage given, reason for administering the medication.
   d. When permission is given to administer medication on an "as needed" basis, the parent must be notified on the same day of the amount administered and the time it was administered.
4. Discipline
   a. The provider shall establish simple, understandable rules so that the expectations and limitations are clear to the child, the parent(s), and to any other care givers.

b. The provider shall not use, or permit another person to use, corporal punishment (i.e., striking, slapping, spanking with a hand or any other instrument), or punishment which is abusive or humiliating.
   c. Food shall not be withheld as a means of punishment, nor shall a child be punished for refusing food.
   d. There shall be no verbal abuse, threats, or derogatory remarks about the child or the child's family.
   e. No child shall be punished for toileting accidents.
5. Program and Care of Children
   a. There shall be activities which provide a variety of experiences geared to the ages and abilities of the child(ren). Activities shall allow choice, and encourage a child to develop skills in all areas appropriate to the child's age and ability. A balance of active and quiet play shall be provided both indoors and outdoors when weather permits.
   b. The program shall provide regularity in routines such as, but not limited to, eating, napping, and toileting, and sufficient flexibility to respond to the needs of the individual.

412–10–436 Administration

1. Exceptions—Exceptions to an individual standard set forth in these rules may be granted for good and just cause by the Division. The provider shall make application in writing to the Division.
2. Enforcement
   a. In order to ascertain compliance with these standards, CSD may inspect at any reasonable time the premises and required records of any registered home.
   b. In some instances there are no common definitions as to degree of acceptability. For these rules the determination of acceptability and of nonacceptability shall be made at the discretion of CSD.
   c. CSD shall not accept a new application for registration for at least one year following the denial of an application or revocation.
   d. Upon failure to meet standards or correct deficiencies,

CSD may deny an application, or revoke, or suspend registration.

e. The provider has the right to appeal any decision to deny, revoke, or suspend subject to the provisions of Chapter 183, Oregon Revised Statutes.

State of Oregon
CHILDREN'S SERVICES DIVISION
Department of Human Resources

INSURANCE: WHY AND HOW

Whether you have one child in your care or five, you will need insurance. This is necessary for your protection. Society has become lawsuit-happy. What was considered an accident and forgotten 10 years ago is now considered by many people a way to get money.

Suppose that Mr. Brown comes to pick up his son Jonathan. It has been raining all day. Mr. Brown gathers Jonathan's belongings and carries them and his son out your door. Suddenly, Mr. Brown slips and falls on your front porch. Both he and little Jonathan appear fine, and go home. That night you receive a phone call for your insurance number. Mr. Brown has injured his back.

If you were not insured, how would you pay Mr. Brown's doctor bills, or his time loss from work? What if Mr. Brown sued you for his injuries? Would you lose your savings, car, or home?

What if a child in your care was severely injured? How would you pay for the hospital bills if the child's parents demanded it? You couldn't if you weren't insured.

How do you insure your day-care business? In most cases, if you are caring for four or fewer children, you can get coverage under your homeowner's policy. This is called an insurance rider, and it is usually very inexpensive.

However, if you are caring for more children than your insurance company will allow on a rider, you will need specialty insurance. This is a business-type insurance, and it is very expensive. A typical day-care specialty insurance policy could cost you the equivalent for your income from caring for one or two children for an entire year. This is substantial, and may help you to decide to limit care to four or fewer full-time children.

It is also necessary to make sure that you carry enough auto insurance. If you are using your car for field trips or picking up and dropping off children, you must be protected. Talk to your insurance agent about liability limits. Each child should be covered for at least $300,000 in liability.

Insurance is a vital expense. You hope you will never have to file a claim. But if something does happen, you will be relieved to know that your insurance will cover it. As a provider, you deserve the peace of mind and protection that insurance can provide.

HOW TO ADVERTISE

Every business needs a way to let people know that it is open, where it is located, and what it offers. As a day-care professional, you will have to let the public know that you are open for business. You will have to advertise exactly what you offer, and when and how it may be obtained.

Before you advertise, you should consider your capability for meeting the needs of a particular group of parents. If you advertise, for instance, on a business bulletin board, you are likely to get parents who work similar schedules.

You must also consider your desires and those of your family. You will have to decide if you want to care for children during the day, during swing shift, or during graveyard shift. You will also have to decide if you want to care for drop-ins or not.

Parents will want your ad to answer their concerns about the quality of care, age groups you accept, and the cost of your services. For instance: Will their child be safe? Will there be activities for their child to enjoy? Will snacks or meals be served? Are you a responsible person? Are you experienced? Do you have references? These are primary concerns for parents seeking day care. Try to answer them in your advertising.

When you are ready to advertise, you will have to decide what to charge for your services. Call local day care centers or the Children's Services Divisions, and inquire about their rates for child care. Check newspaper ads to determine an acceptable fee. You can even call other local providers to ask about their rates. Make sure that you identify yourself as a new provider when calling. Do not pretend to be a parent inquiring about their services. This is not fair to the other provider. You should be able to determine what a fair charge is for your services in a relatively short time.

You need to determine the advantages and disadvantages of your location, too. Then, consider your values and principles. Ask yourself the following questions. They will help prepare you to answer inquiries from parents who are replying to your ad.

1. What hours will I care for children?
2. How many children will I accept for care?
3. Will I only accept children whose parents have similar values?
4. What ages of children will I accept?
5. Do I have a school nearby?
6. Do I live close to a park?
7. If I care for more than one child from a single family, will I reduce my fee?
8. Is my home easy to find?
9. If I smoke, am I prepared to inform parents?
10. How many other people are in my home?
11. Do I have references?
12. Am I willing to accept children whose parents do not value cleanliness in the same manner as I do?
13. Am I prepared to inform parents of my religious or ethnic practices?
14. Does my home have a fenced yard?
15. Is my home suitable for infants? Preschoolers? Children with handicaps?

After answering these questions, you are ready to write your ad. Make sure that your statements are clear, easy to understand, and concise. Include enough information to draw attention. Don't try to explain all of your services. Your ad should arouse interest, thereby stimulating the parents to inquire further. Always include your phone number, but not your address. You want the reader to phone first, so that you can screen out undesirable respondents.

There are three inexpensive methods of advertising. These are word of mouth, local newspapers, and posters or notices placed in public locations.

If you decide to advertise by word of mouth, allow plenty of time. Visit your local schools to let their officials know that you are beginning a day-care business. They often receive requests from parents for child care persons. Tell all of your friends, and ask them to spread the word. This may make for a slow start, but it costs nothing financially.

On the other hand, advertising in the newspaper can be expensive. You ad must be shorter, and you have no control over who may answer it. If you advertise in weekly shoppers, the cost will be less expensive. You will also reach your local community.

You may decide to make posters. You can include more information this way. Use bold letters to attract attention. Avoid being too cute. Parents may feel that you are not serious enough in your attitude. Ask permission to put up your poster. Doctors' or dentists' offices are good places to start. You might also try grocery stores and businesses. Consider posting a small tear-off pad with your phone number and brief information on each page. This will allow parents to take your number with them.

Whatever method of advertising you decide on will produce some results. It may take time to open your business with that first child, but before you know it you will be off to a start. If one method does not work at first, try another. Be persistent. Anything worth having is worth the effort it takes to build it. Your day-care business is a valuable service to your community. Don't get discouraged. Just keep on advertising!

PARENT INTERVIEWS

Some time has passed since you began advertising your day-care business. You begin to receive phone calls from interested and prospective parents. How can you determine if the parents phoning are those you may want to meet?

It is possible to screen all prospective parents before you make an appointment to meet them. Even though the callers will ask you question after question, your own questions must be answered too. There are six basic questions to ask each prospective parent before making an appointment to meet them.

1. How old is your child?
2. Has your child been in day care before?
3. Does your child have any special medical or personal problems?
4. How long have you been employed? And what is your occupation?
5. What do you expect from a day-care provider?
6. Do you have two personal references? If the child has been in previous care, ask for the name of the last provider.

Listen carefully to each answer. Write it down, and your own impressions. Ask them for their phone number so you can call them back in a half hour to set up an appointment.

Once you are off the phone, immediately check their references, especially the last day-care provider. Ask about the parents' reliability. Find out what their child is like. As if they paid on time. If you have a providers' organization in your area, call them to find out if the prospective parents have been put on a nonpayment list.

After you have reviewed the basic information you have collected, decided if you would like to make an appointment or not. If you decide not to, telephone them at once. Let them know that you feel you are not suited to meet their requirements. If they ask why you feel that way, tell them as honestly and tactfully as possible. Be honest, making sure that they do not get the impression that any form of prejudice is involved. Be polite and firm.

Once you have decided to make an appointment, arrange it with them. Ask that the child not come with them for the first visit. Explain that you would like to get to know them better before meeting the child. This will safeguard you from accepting a child who is appealing when you have questions about the parents. You must develop a relationship with the parents as well as the child.

When the prospective parents arrive, show them the areas of your home used for your business. Then discuss fully your home rules: hours you are available, fees charged, method of payment required, and what you will tolerate and what you won't. Answer all of their questions completely, too.

When the initial interview is over, arrange for the parents to return with their child. After the parents leave, review the data. Were their personalities compatible with yours? Did they respect you as a professional? What was their general demeanor? Where are they employed? Review everything about them before your second visit. Remember that all families do not fit neatly into one package. The preconceived idea of a conventional family, with Daddy, Mommy, Dick, and Jane, is outdated. In an increasing number of families, a single parent acts as head of the household. Boyfriends or girlfriends, stepmothers or stepfathers may pick up or drop off the children. When considering caring for a child do not allow the family's structure to be the determining factor.

On the follow-up visit, observe their child carefully. Ask yourself if this is a child you could relate to. Notice how the parents and the child interact. Is it apparent that the child is well-adjusted and secure? Will their child fit into your day-care routine?

At the end of the visit decide if you will take the child or not. If not, tell the parents that you feel that you are not best suited to meet the child's specific needs. These needs could include length of time in care, feeding or sleeping schedule, and the amount of attention he will require. If you decide to accept the child, explain that you will do so for a trial period of one month. This will allow you to change your mind if the situation does not live up to your expectations. When this occurs, explain to the parents that your day care is made up of the personalities of many children. It is your responsibility to determine which children will keep the environment running smoothly. Your decision should not imply that the child is inferior, just that his needs cannot be met by your program.

Give the parents an admission information form and a let's-get-acquainted form. Instruct them to fill them out completely before they leave. Establish a starting date and inform them as to what they are to provide on a daily basis. You are now in business!

AGREEMENTS, CONTRACTS, AND CHILDREN'S RECORDS

As a day-care provider, it is necessary for you to maintain certain records concerning your day-care children. Three such records are parent agreements, parent contracts, and children's records.

The Agreement

The agreement, which is between you and the parent, must include what you agree to provide in services. Many providers write this in letter form to their day-care parents ("letter of agreement").

When writing your agreement, think about what you will be offering and what you will not. For instance, will you provide *all* meals for your day-care children? If you provide *some*, be specific about which meals you will be serving. Write down exactly the number of meals and snacks to be served on a daily basis.

Also include all supplies the parents are expected to provide. If you want them to bring a change of clothing, diapers, or extra bottles, include those requirements in your agreement. You may also want to include particulars of dress and grooming. For instance, even with sandals, socks are to be worn. Specifics now can avert problems later.

The parent agreement is also the place to specify your requirements for ill children. Include what you expect to be paid if children do not come on non-vacation days. State length, and if possible, dates, of your vacation, as well as the amount of notice to be given before you take time off.

After you have written your agreement, reread it to make sure all aspects of your requirements have been included. Your final paragraph should discuss your termination policy. If you require parents to give you a 2-week notice before terminating your services, write it down. This will protect you, somewhat, from parents calling the night before to cancel.

Have the parents sign and date the agreement. You must sign it too. Then give them a copy maintaining the original for your records. This then becomes a legal document. If a parent fails to live up to the agreement, you have legal reasons to discharge them or cancel your services. It will also be important if you have to go to small claims court for parental nonpayment. An example of a parent agreement is found in Chapter 8 under Sample Forms.

The Contract

The contract is much briefer than the parent agreement. It simply contains the information pertinent to your business: the days the child is to be in your care, the time period, rate of pay, method of payment, and any late fees.

You can make up your own contract, or you can purchase a standard one from an office supply store. A sample contract is offered in Chapter 8.

The importance of a contract cannot be overstressed. Without it, you have almost no way of obtaining fees from nonpaying parents.

Have the parent (if possible, both parents) sign and date the contract. After they have signed it, add your signature. Give the parents a carbon copy, and keep the original in your record files.

Children's Records

Your day-care business will require you to maintain certain records on the children in your care. You will need records for your own information as well as for the parents'. In case of a medical emergency you will also need records regarding the child's medical history.

Maintaining children's records will provide you with information concerning the needs of the child. If will also protect you from possible misunderstanding between yourself and a parent. You will be ready to meet a medical emergency, and you will have authorization to seek medical help. Records act as a provider/parent communication system, and give both you and the parent peace of mind.

Parents feel secure because they are assured that you are organized and ready to meet the needs of their child. It also gives them the opportunity to contribute essential information for the well-being of their child.

This system also benefits the child, who will feel comfortable and confident when there is clear agreement between their parents and their care giver. The children's needs will also be easier to meet when you know exactly what the needs are.

Keeping the necessary records on each child in your care does not have to be complicated. It just requires basic organization. The easiest way is to keep a folder for each child. You can put all pertinent information in the folder, and then file the folder for easy access.

In case of a medical emergency, you will need a parent permission form to take with you to the hospital. Keep this form along with the child's medical history and list of allergies in a separate folder. This folder can be distinctly marked, so you can pull it quickly when needed.

What type of records do you need to maintain on each child?

1. Admission form: This provides all pertinent information such as birthdate, full name, parents' names, parents' places of business, emergency phone numbers, etc.
2. Authorization form: This is the parent's permission for you to seek emergency medical aid.
3. Medical history: allergies, vaccinations, doctor's name, insurance numbers, and any related medical problems are included.
4. Parent agreement
5. Parent contract
6. Attendance record: this records when the child is in your care—days and hours.
7. Permission to administer drugs: parents must sign this each time you are to give their child medication. They are also to record the amounts. If a certain drug is to be given on an "as needed" basis, have the parent write that down, too.

8. Illness record: Write down the date and time a child becomes ill while in your care. Also include when you notified the parent and the treatment you administered. If the child has, or has had, a communicable disease, write it down, too.
9. Record of injuries: This is to record any injury a child receives in your home. It must be included even if it seems minor. Notify the parents of every injury.

SCHEDULING YOUR DAY

Is it possible for you to keep your day on an even keel? If you set a basic schedule to follow, you will be able to. It may require an extra effort, but an efficient schedule is directly related to how successfully you manage your time.

When providing care for several small children, you will have to schedule mealtimes, nap times, craft activities, outdoor play, as well as potty training. You will also be required to cook, clean, launder, and take care of your own family's needs. Therefore, in order to accomplish all daily tasks, and keep your sanity, you need to use your time wisely. A sound daily schedule will aid you in this endeavor.

The first thing to consider is what hours you will be caring for children. Then write down the times that your family will be coming and going. Be sure to include family mealtimes. You will probably already notice conflicts. For instance, your day-care children begin arriving at 6:30 a.m. Your spouse has to leave for work at 7 a.m. You must serve your spouse's breakfast and pack the lunch. Then your children must get out of bed and get ready for school. They must eat and leave with lunches in hand at 8:30 a.m. In the meantime, you have had three hungry day-care children arrive at three different times. How do you possibly cover all bases?

First of all, you must get help from your family. Secondly, you must work out a schedule that is the easiest for you. Example: pack and refrigerate lunches the night before, set the breakfast table the night before; try to arrange for all children to eat breakfast together. It is your decision as to what your priorities will be. List them on your schedule.

Perhaps the easiest items to schedule will be meals, snacks, and naps. Write down these times and plan to stick to this schedule until it becomes a natural routine.

It is impossible to schedule all of your day. There will always be minor and major crises. This is why your schedule must be somewhat flexible. If you expect everything to happen right on time, you are going to feel pressured. Children need routine to feel secure. At the same time, though, they are great schedule-benders. Stephanie may be tired at 11 a.m. while Jamie may refuse to take a nap till it's time to go home. All mishaps must be taken in stride. If you expect the unexpected, you will not become discouraged.

A basic schedule will not only make your day run more smoothly, it will give you a professional attitude about yourself and your business.

Chapter 3

RECORDS TO KEEP FOR TAXES

The idea of maintaining the appropriate records for tax purposes can be intimidating. Yet, the law requires a day-care provider to file a tax return. How can you prepare yourself to handle the record-keeping tasks that are demanded of your profession?

In order to know exactly what is required, as far as record-keeping goes, you must know the IRS guidelines. The Internal Revenue Service offers a publication, *Business Use of Your Home*, updated each year as the tax laws change. You can get a copy of this pamphlet by telephoning your local IRS office. They will mail you the revised edition, but allow a few weeks for delivery. Although the IRS updates its tax information annually, the guidelines given are relatively standard. They will enable you to understand what is required so that an accurate record-keeping system can be established. The facts given cannot relieve you of the responsibility for acquiring the revised yearly guidelines. Each professional is responsible for himself.

IRS GUIDELINES

If you use part of your home in your business, you can deduct certain expenses for this use. The Internal Revenue Service requires that businesses meet specific tests, and often your deduction is limited.

Generally, whether you are an employee or a self-employed person, you may not deduct expenses for the business use of your home. This general rule does not apply if the use of your home meets specific business requirements. The following information is based on the 1985 *Business Use of Your Home* provided by the IRS.

Use tests

In order to take a deduction for using part of your home in business, that part of your home must be used exclusively and regularly as:

1. The principal place of business for any trade or business in which you engage.
2. A place to meet or deal with your patients, clients, or customers in the normal course of your trade or business.
3. In connection with your trade or business, if you are using a separate structure that is not attached to your house or residence.

"Exclusive use" means that you must use a specific part of your home only for the purpose of carrying on your trade or business. If you use part of your home as your business office and also use it for personal purposes, you have not met the "exclusive use" test.

However, there are two exceptions to the "exclusive use" test. The use of part of your home for the storage of inventory is the first exception. The second exception is the use of your home, or part of it, as a day-care facility.

When part of your home is used as a day-care facility on a regular basis, you may deduct expenses incurred: if, that is, you can meet the following requirements that have been established by the IRS.

1. You must be in the trade of business of providing day care for children, for persons 65 or older, or for persons who are physically or mentally unable to care for themselves.
2. The owner or operator of the day-care business must have applied for, been granted, or be exempt from having a license, certification, registration, or approval as a day-care center or as a family or group day-care home under any applicable state law. This requirement is not met if the application has been rejected or the license or other authorization has been revoked.

"Regular use" means that you use the exclusively business part of your home on a continuing basis. Occasional or incidental use does not meet the test. This rule applies even if a specific part of your home is used for no other purpose. You must be in family day care as a business in order to meet these qualifications. You can not just occasionally care for a child or two and expect to take deductions for a home business.

Figuring deductions

After considering the requirements that have been discussed, your next step is to divide the expenses of operating your home between the business use and the personal use. Certain expenses you will find totally deductible while others are not. The total expenses that you can deduct for the business use of your home cannot exceed the gross income from your day-care business. Nor can an excess amount of deductions be carried over to the next year.

To clarify: suppose that your gross income from your home day-care business is $3,000, and your allowable deductions come to $3,600. By subtracting your gross income from the amount of your deductions you find that you have a credit of $600. The amount cannot be deducted from your spouse's gross income from another business, nor can it be carried over to the next year to be deducted from that year's gross income. The excess amount cannot be claimed in any way.

You do derive a benefit from the excess amount, however. It is not a financial gain, but it is of value to you. You gain the knowledge that if your deductions remain the same in the following year, you can increase your gross income by that $600 and not owe any extra tax. This knowledge may lead to you add one more child to your day-care home. The earnings will increase your gross income, but the care of that child will probably increase the amount of your allowable deductions too.

How do you divide each expense and figure your total deduction? In order to do this properly you must retain records that provide the information that is needed to figure your deduction. You should keep all cancelled checks, receipts, and other evidence of the expenses you paid. You must be able to show:

1. The part of your home that you use for business.
2. That you use this part of your home according to the exclusive and regular use tests as your principal place of business.
3. The amount of depreciation and other expenses for keeping up your home that are for business use.

Business part. To figure the part of your home used for business can be very difficult for the day-care provider. Most providers use their entire home for their day-care children. If you use a specific area, however, such as only the basement, you must measure the area in square feet. If the rooms are about the same size, you may figure this part by dividing the number of rooms used for business by the number of rooms in the home.

For example: you use one room for your business that measures 120 square feet. You are therefore, using one tenth (120/1,200), or 10 percent of the total area for business. If the rooms in your home are equivalent in size and you use one room for business in a 5- room house, you are using one-fifth, or 20 percent, of the total area for business.

In a day-care home, you must also figure the percentage of use. This is done by keeping accurate records regarding the hours you have children in care. There are 8,760 hours in the year. If you provide day care in your home for 2,920 hours, your home has been in business use for one-third or 33 percent of the year. This percentage will vary from provider to provider. The figures that you arrive at for the percentage of use will be valuable when calculating expenses relating to the use of your home for your day-care business.

EXPENSES AND DEDUCTIONS

Your earnings from your home day-care business are taxable income. In order to determine what part of your income is taxable, you must figure your net profit. This is the amount that remains after subtracting from the gross profit the expenses you incurred in the operation of your business. The net profit is the amount that is then subject to income tax, not the amount that was paid to you for providing child care. The value of identifying and recording all related expenses is thus shown. There are two types of expenses that must be considered: direct and indirect.

Direct Expenses

Direct expenses are expenditures of cash that benefit only the business part of your home. They include painting or repairs made in the specific area or room that is used for your business. Expenditures that are part of a general plan to recondition, improve, or alter your house to make it suitable are classified under capital expenditures. A capital expenditure is an investment of capital in property that has a useful life of more than 1 year or that is a permanent improvement to the property This would increase the value of the property, add to its life, or give it a new or different use. Examples of such improvements would include rewiring, plumbing, new roof, etc. If, however, you repaired the roof instead of replacing it with a new roof, the expense would be a direct expense.

As a day-care provider, the expenses directly related to the business use of your home are not fully deductible. These are subject to deduction limitation. You are aware that your total deduction for business use of your home cannot exceed your gross income. You must first subtract the business part of your real estate taxes, mortgage interest, and casualty losses from this gross income. If the business part of these deductions is more than your business gross income, you cannot deduct any of your other expenses for the business use of your home. Although you may deduct all of your real estate taxes, mortgage interest, and casualty losses as itemized deductions, you must still use the business part of these items to figure the limit on your total deductions for the business use of your home according to the IRS.

After subtracting the business expenses from your deductions for real estate taxes, mortgage interest, and casualty losses you may deduct, first, operating expenses, and then depreciation of property.

Operating expenses will vary from provider to provider. These will include all actual day-care expenses that you incur because you are caring for children. There are many possibilities. Some are:

1. food
2. crayons, paints, and craft supplies
3. glue
4. paper
5. toys
6. bottles
7. diapers
8. books
9. records and tapes
10. sleeping equipment
11. cleaning supplies
12. repairs
13. advertising
14. postage
15. office supplies
16. backup care
17. entertainment
18. computer games
19. movie VCR rentals
20. sports equipment
21. board games
22. crafts, dance, or music classes outside the day-care home
23. insurance
24. clothing for children

25. bad debts
26. linens
27. musical instruments

After you have determined what your direct expenses are, make sure that you maintain accurate records of each one. Save your sales receipts from each purchase. You will need to show them to the IRS if your tax return is audited. Since the IRS can examine a tax return up to 3 years after it is filed, it is very important to keep all receipts as proof of each expense claimed for that time period.

If the receipt is not computerized, write the name of the item purchased next to the amount. Then write the amount of the direct expense on your monthly expense record. Include the date, amount, and a brief description of the item purchased. Do this as soon as possible. Do not allow yourself to put off recording each expense as it occurs. Otherwise you will find that you have misplaced or lost some receipts, or you may have forgotten what was purchased and when. This can mean fewer deductions to subtract from your gross income, and more taxes to pay on a larger net profit.

Food Expense

There is one direct expense that can cause much confusion. This is the cost of supplying food to your day-care children. If you actually buy different food for the children and keep it separate from your family's food, you can simply save the cash register tapes and list them on your expense record.

If you usually serve the same food to your family and your day-care children, then you must find a method of recording the expense. Two such methods are:

1. Keep a record of all your food expenses each month. Figure what percentage of the food was served to the day-care children. Then multiply the total food expense by the percentage used by the children.
2. Decide on a reasonable average cost for the food you serve the children each day. Multiply that average cost by the

number of children in care, and then by the number of days.

Each method mentioned has its drawbacks. The first requires heavy record keeping. It also is very difficult to determine what percentage of food is used by your day-care children. For instance, how do you determine the percentage of food eaten by two preschoolers when you have three teenagers and two adults eating the same food. The more children in your care, the more confusing it becomes.

The second method may be the most practical one to follow. You will have to show that your estimate of the cost of the food you serve per day is reasonable. You might accomplish this by buying food for your day-care children separately from your family food for several weeks. Keep an accurate record of the cost and numbers of children fed. This will prove that your average daily food cost per child is reasonable.

Another way to use this method is to refer to the USDA Standard Food Cost Factors. The USDA has established specific food costs for each meal and snack eaten by children. It is according to this established amount that the USDA offers food cost reimbursement. Day-care providers who are enrolled in the USDA program are reimbursed for three meals or snacks each day that are served to the day-care children. In return the provider agrees to supply nutritious meals that meet USDA requirements. You must also maintain monthly menus that are submitted to the sponsoring agency for the USDA reimbursement. Contact a family day-care support system to get the current figures.

The USDA food program will pay you extra money for serving meals that meet certain nutritional requirements. You must keep careful records of each check you receive. Include the amount on your monthly income record. The total amount received must be added as income to your annual gross income. On your monthly expense record include the total amount for each meal and snack served. Since USDA only pays for three meals or snacks, the amount in your expense column will always be greater than the amount you received from USDA. This will total a sizeable food expense at the end of the year, especially when you consider that most day-care children eat at least two meals and two snacks each day they are in care.

Indirect expenses

Indirect expenses are those that benefit the day-care children and your family. These include expenses that you would normally have, but which may be higher because of your home day-care business. An indirect expense must be related in some way to the part of your home used for your business. The business part of these expenses is deductible.

Examples of indirect expenses are:

1. real estate taxes
2. mortgage interest
3. casualty losses
4. rent
5. utilities
6. insurance
7. major repairs
8. depreciation

You will need to figure the percentage of your home that is used by your day-care business in order to determine the business part of your indirect expenses. For instance, if you use all of your home for day care and have children in your home 25 percent of the time, then you may deduct 25 percent of all indirect expenses. Check with the IRS to verify the amount that may be deducted as indirect expenses.

When figuring your deductions carefully, review Publication #583, *Information for Business Taxpayers*, and Publication #587, *Business Use of Your Home*. As previously mentioned, the publications are available free upon request from the Internal Revenue Service. If any point is still unclear, ask the IRS for help. The preparer may not be aware of the expenses that can occur in a home day-care business. You need to be precise and informative when speaking with any tax preparer.

SOCIAL SECURITY AND SELF-EMPLOYMENT TAX

Day-care providers are considered self-employed persons by the Internal Revenue Service. As such you must pay self-employment tax, or as it is commonly referred to, Social Security. If your net profit exceeds $400 per year, you are required to pay 7.05 percent of your wages up to $39,600 (1985).

You will need to call your local IRS office in order to have the proper reporting forms sent to your home. They will also send information on how to complete them and when to file them. Failure to report your income may result in a penalty that must be paid in addition to the overdue taxes.

Remember that you are required to base your Social Security payments on your net profit, not your gross income. Your net profit can be determined on a monthly basis through your day-care income and expense records. Carefully review each month's records. If it appears that after deducting your expenses from your gross income your net profit exceeds $400, report it without delay.

You may elect to make quarterly reports if it appears that your estimated Social Security tax for the year exceeds $500. A calendar quarter is a 3-month period that ends on March 31, June 30, September 30, or December 31. Within a month after a quarter ends, you are required to send your tax and reporting form to the Internal Revenue Service.

Since day-care providers are by no means independently wealthy, and require every dollar to meet daily needs, you may question the value of reporting your net profit. Social Security, however, is much more than a retirement program. It also pays monthly benefits to the worker or the worker's dependents if she becomes disabled for a year or more. If a worker dies, her dependents may receive payments.

In order to receive such benefits, you must build up Social Security credits. In 1985, a person earned one quarter of coverage for every $410 of reported annual earnings. This is up to a maximum of four quarters for the year. Failure to report your "net profit" and to make your required Social Security, or self-employment tax payment will limit the amount of protection you will receive from Social Security. It will also mean that penalties will be levied against you. Take steps to make sure that your day-care business reports all "net profits" exceeding $400 to the Internal Revenue Service.

ESTABLISHING AN EASY BOOKKEEPING SYSTEM

Congratulations! You have established your very own home day-care business. So far, you have had to make tremendous adjustments, for your own part, and for your family. You have made the changes that have been demanded of you. Now you must develop a system for keeping track of money earned and how it is spent. The importance of maintaining accurate records can not be overstressed.

When you have a business in your home, you need to prove income and its source. You are required to file a tax return on your earned income at tax time. The appropriate records can enable this to go smoothly. A well set up bookkeeping system will not only make it easier to prepare your taxes, but it will also back up the figures you put on your tax form. The Internal Revenue Service requires that you prove every figure on your return. How do you establish such a system?

Make an appointment with a tax consultant to determine what your state and the IRS require. Then review Chapter 8 of this book. You will find sample bookkeeping forms for home day care. With the help of your tax consultant determine which forms will be included in your bookkeeping system. The following is a list of suggested forms and descriptions of their possible use. You will have to modify the forms to meet your own requirements. They are as follows:

1. Day-Care Attendance Record
2. Meals Served Report
3. Parent Payment Record
4. Monthly Expense Record
5. Annual Income and Expense
6. Yearly Tally Sheet
7. Monthly Mileage Auto Record
8. Home Computer Use
9. Equipment Use

The day-care attendance record can be used weekly or monthly. You must be able to prove to the IRS and to parents what days and hours you cared for the children. Maintaining this record will help you to determine the hourly use of your home for your day-care business. This is vital in figuring your indirect expenses. It is also necessary in collecting your fee from the children's parents. One glance will tell both of you exactly what days a particular child was in your care.

If you plan on serving meals and snacks to your day-care children, you will need to keep track of each one. To qualify for an income tax deduction, you must record each meal served. If you are on the USDA food program, you are required to file an attendance record with your menu. You will need to maintain a record in your bookkeeping system of the meals served. Remember, USDA only reimburses for three meals a day. Since most day-care children receive two meals and two snacks daily, one meal can qualify as a day-care expense.

The parent payment record is very important. This record allows you to verify your income. It also makes you aware of nonpayment for your services. Carefully record each payment. You can use one sheet for each child in care.

Income and expense records can be used to record income received and expenses incurred on a monthly basis. If the forms are not complete enough for you, invest in a 10-column bookkeeping record. These are available at your local office supply outlet. You can use one sheet for each month. The 10 columns allow you to add any expenses that you may have. For example, you might include: laundry, cleaning supplies, advertising, insurance, paper supplies, postage, legal fees, toys, books, etc. By using a monthly expense and income record you can easily tally both at year's end.

If you use your automobile with your day-care children, you must keep accurate mileage records. You might want to purchase an auto record. This can be kept in the car for recording purposes. Then each time that you drive your day-care children somewhere, write down your beginning mileage. When you return, record your ending mileage. Record the total miles driven and the purpose for the auto's use. If you use your car often, say, to pick up and deliver children, then this simple task can provide you with a substantial deduction on your income tax.

Some providers equip their homes with computers, VCRs, televisions, and other instruments. If you make such equipment available to your day-care children, you are required to record its use. You must log personal use and business use to determine the percentage of the deduction allowed. Ask your tax consultant what is required each year. As mentioned before, the tax laws change every year. One year you may be required to record equipment usage, the next year you may not. Take the time to verify the changes in the tax laws. This will keep your bookkeeping system accurate.

After you have assembled your records into an easily maintained system, you may also want to add some large manila envelopes. It's a good idea to use one for each month. Use the manila envelopes to store your monthly receipts. This simple step will keep you organized. No more lost receipts at tax time either. You can even number each receipt to correspond to a numbered entry on your expense record. Then if you are asked to produce your receipt for a specific expense, you will be able to find it quickly.

Keeping the appropriate records can be time-consuming. But, by doing so you will always know where your money has gone. You will be aware of each expense and will be able to prove each deduction taken. Your home day care is a business, and as its ower you are required to maintain the appropriate records. Doing so will help make your business profitable and enjoyable.

Chapter 4

MEAL PLANNING

Now that you have children in your care, what do you feed them? After all, day-care providers usually care for young children from 8 to 10 hours a day. This means that the children in a provider's care will eat more meals there than at the parent's home. This puts a great responsibility on the provider to plan and serve nutritious meals.

GOOD NUTRITION

Children need good nutrition in the form of well-balanced meals, to grow physically, mentally, and emotionally. The food you serve will furnish all the building materials the children in your care need for growth, health, and energy. Protein and minerals are needed for growing, building, and repairing body tissue, muscles, and bones. Vitamins will help to protect the body and keep it functioning well. Fuel for activity is provided by fats and carbohydrates. No one food can provide all of these elements. You must prepare a wide variety of foods from the four basic food groups in order to give your day-care children sound nutrition.

Good food habits

Healthy children generally have good appetites. They know when they are hungry and when they have had enough to eat. How much they eat will vary from day to day. Many factors, such as rate of growth, activity, and sense of well-being will influence how much they eat. To promote a good appetite try to serve meals at regular times and encourage active outside play. Never force children to eat. By helping your day-care children to develop good food habits while they are in your care, you are giving them good food habits that will last a lifetime.

Serve child-size portions at mealtimes with the understanding that seconds are available. The amount of food children will consume depends on their age, size, growth, and amount of activity. If a child refuses to eat, avoid making an issue out of it. Encourage the children to try new foods before they pass judgment on them. Again, this will develop good eating habits.

Learning experience. Food can provide a favorable learning experience in day care. If children are to learn to like food, they must enjoy it. Food likes and dislikes are mostly learned reactions. Children learn to desire certain foods through repetition and imitation. Introduce new foods in small amounts. Be positive, and assume that the children will like the new food, but don't make an issue of their not eating it. Allow your day-care children to help you in preparing meals. This will help to promote good feelings about the food. Small children especially enjoy stirring, kneading, and just about anything they can do with their hands. Older children can help make simple puddings, sandwiches, salads, and cookies.

Food problems

What if, after all your efforts to develop good food habits, some of your day-care children develop food problems? How do you handle a child who refuses to eat, a dawdler, or a child who goes on a food jag? Basically, you don't make an issue of it. Most children will refuse to eat occasionally. Perhaps they ate a snack shortly before mealtime. Maybe they are simply asserting their independence, or they may just not feel hungry. Relax; do not force them to eat. Let their parent know about the problem, and how you are handling it. A healthy child will survive a missed meal without ill effect.

The dawdler is another problem day-care providers face. You can have as few as two children, or as many as six, and be thankful if you only have one dawdler in the bunch. Some dawdling is always expected; but a child who takes three times as long as the others holds up schedule—especially, if the dawdler is just finishing lunch when afternoon snack is ready for the other children. What can you do? Don't make an issue of it! If the child is tired, maybe you could help with the rest of the meal. Perhaps the child has a short attention span and quickly loses interest in the food. If this is the case, try adding a few extra touches. For instance, a plain canned pear can become a bunny by adding some raisins for eyes and carrots strips for ears. Check the following recipes to make food fun. Dawdling may also be a ploy to get attention. Ignoring the situation and refusing to get upset over it will soon put an end to the dawdling game.

The child on a food jag is especially trying. What do you do if all the child will eat are peanut butter and jelly sandwiches? No matter how you cajole the child, peanut butter and jelly wins. Be careful not to enter a battle of wills. Chances are that the child will never give in. So you might as well let them enjoy their peanut butter and jelly sandwiches. Talk with the child's parents about the problem in the child's absence. Together, maybe you can come up with an answer. Probably, though, about the time you find a solution the child will be hooked on bananas and yogurt. Whatever happens, try not to make an issue of it and it will pass.

USDA GUIDELINES

The USDA food program was created by the Department of Agriculture to provide training and assistance to day-care providers in order that nutritionally balanced meals be served to the children of working parents.

Day-care providers are offered reimbursement for day-care

food costs. In order to qualify for these funds you must keep accurate records of the foods served and to whom they are served. You must also be licensed to provide day care. Every meal or snack you serve must follow specific food requirements. These requirements not only cover what types of food you may serve but also what amounts must be served for each age group.

The basic USDA guidelines are as follows:
Breakfast:

>   vegetable, fruit, or juice
>   cereal, bread, or bread alternate
>   fluid milk (any but powdered milk or reconstituted dry milk)

Mid-morning:

>   meat or meat alternate
>   vegetable, fruit, or juice*
>   enriched or whole grain bread, or bread alternate
>   fluid milk*

*Two liquids may not be served together to meet snack requirements.

Do not serve two foods from the same food group.
Lunch or supper:

>   meat or meat alternate
>   two or more vegetables or fruits
>   enriched or whole grain bread, or bread alternate
>   fluid milk

Certain foods are restricted in credit allowances for the USDA food program. Some of these are potato chips, popcorn, nuts, bacon, cream cheese, gelatin Jell-O, coconut, yogurt, and tofu. These foods are considered to either be too high in salt and fat content or do not supply the necessary nutrients needed by young children.

Under the meat heading are also found meat alternates. These include beans or peas, cheese, cheese foods (amounts to be used increase), chicken, fish sticks, tuna, peanut butter, and eggs. Hot dogs, sausage, and bologna can be used, but if they contain sodium nitrates they are not recommended. You are advised to read the label on such products.

Fresh milk is required at breakfast, lunch, and supper as a fluid. When serving juices you are required to serve only those that are fresh, frozen, or canned, 100 percent pure juice. These include orange, pineapple, prune, apple, grape, grapefruit/orange, tangerine, tomato, and lemon. Drinks such as Kool-Aid, Tang, Hi-C, or any so-called cocktail, drink, ade, base, nectar, or punch are not acceptable. Again, check the label to find out if it is allowed.

The acceptable bread or bread alternate group is quite extensive. Basically any product that is made of whole grain or enriched flour or meal is acceptable. Products that are not acceptable are in two groups. The first are sweet-type foods such as cakes and pies that are usually served for dessert. The exceptions to this rule are cookies. A three- to six-year-old child may be served 17.5 grams of cookie at snack time. The second group includes snack type foods such as hard, thin pretzels, corn chips, and other extruded and/or shaped items made from grain.

For information on the amounts of food to be served for each age group, please refer to the following weekly menus for infants and children. The amounts suggested are not unreasonable and children do not have to finish every ounce before you get credit. Children must be served the outlined amounts. Sometimes they will want more and sometimes they will want less. It depends on the child. An example of amounts is ½ cup of milk required for one- to three-year-olds; ¾ cup for three- to six-year-olds, and 1 cup for six- to twelve-year-olds.

It may seem that the USDA food program requires a lot of work. Actually it only requires a few minutes for each day. You simply fill out a menu sheet in advance. Then you serve the meals and snacks that you have planned. Fill in the number of children you served. At the end of each month you send in the filled out menu sheets and an attendance record to the sponsoring agency that you belong to. Within a few weeks you will reslice for the last group. Contact your local USDA program for the entire list of recommended amounts.

FOOD FOR FUN

Breakfast

Breakfast is the most often skipped meal of the day. This is unfortunate, because it is also the most important meal. The body has gone for 10 to 12 hours without a replenishment of nutrients. Breakfast provides the necessary nutrients the body needs to get through the day. Ideally, this meal will include fiber, vegetables or fruit, and protein.

Fiber is needed to add roughage to the diet. Roughage keeps the intestines healthy, and in the proper working condition. Whole grains in the form of cereals or bread products fill the need for fiber. They are also important sources of the B vitamins and iron. The B vitamins help the body to grow at a normal rate. Iron helps build healthy blood.

Vegetable or fruit products provide necessary vitamins and minerals the body needs for energy. They are a good source of vitamin A, vitamin C, and fiber. Vitamin A keeps the skin healthy and protects against night blindness. Young children need vitamin A to help their bodies grow properly. Vitamin C builds the material that connects the body cells. It also helps the body to resist infection, and to keep your gums healthy. Fiber, again, is needed to prevent constipation, but it also helps to prevent some diseases of the large intestines. Different fruits and vegetables will give different amounts of these nutrients; so it is a good idea to vary the ones you serve to your day-care children.

Milk is the most widely used source of protein at breakfast. It is required in order for the breakfast you serve to be acceptable to the USDA food program. Milk supplies not only protein for energy, but also calcium which builds strong bones and teeth. Most milk you buy has vitamin D added. This vitamin is needed to help the body absorb the calcium that it requires.

Serving a good breakfast doesn't have to be time-consuming. It can be as simple as orange wedges, toasted English muffin, and milk. The important point is to choose the elements of a balanced breakfast.

Eating breakfast can be fun. Allow your day-care children to help in preparing it. They will appreciate it more. It will prove to be a nice time to spend together, and a cheery way to begin a new day. Recipes have been included for your convenience. Feel free to change them to suit your taste. Experiment with your own new ideas to make breakfast fun for you and your day-care children.

Breakfast Ideas

1. orange julius
   whole wheat crackers
2. cheese toast
   tangerine
   milk
3. pineapple
   rye toast
   milk
4. tomato juice
   leftover chicken
   milk
5. fruit milkshake
   whole wheat toast
6. cottage cheese
   rye toast
   milk
7. spiced apple slices
   cornbread
   milk
8. banana
   ready-to-eat cereal
   milk
9. strawberry shake
   bran muffin
10. melon
    biscuits
    milk
11. orange slices
    bagel
    milk
12. strawberries
    English muffin
    milk
13. waffles with pear sauce
    milk
14. raisins
    oatmeal
    milk

Breakfast Fun

Egg Surprise

1 slice bread for each child
1 egg for each child

Allow children to cut center of bread out, with cookie cutter, place in skillet with enough butter to cover bottom of skillet. Break egg into hole and cook on both sides. Top with toasted cut-out.

Scrambled Eggs with Rice

1 egg for each child
½ cup cooked rice per child.

Scramble eggs and add rice. Heat rice thoroughly. Serve.

Animal French Toast

2 pieces of bread per child

Allow children to roll bread out with rolling pin. Cut shapes with cookie cutters (bunnies, horses, dogs, etc.) (Save scraps to make bread crumbs.) Then dip into batter of:

2 eggs, beaten
1 cup milk
1 tsp. cinnamon

Fry on both sides in skillet. Serve at once.

Syrup

Heat applesauce, strawberries, or blueberries. Add a touch of honey and enough water to thin slightly. Serve warm over pancakes or waffles.

Whole Wheat Pancakes
(serves 4–6)

¾ cup whole wheat flour
¾ cup white flour
½ tsp. salt
½ cup nonfat dry milk

Put into large bowl and mix well.

1 egg
1¼ cup water
3 tbsp. oil

Beat egg and add water and oil. Then beat until mixed. Mix liquid ingredients into dry ingredients. Stir only until mixed. The batter will be lumpy. Cook on lightly greased hot griddle. Turn over when bubbles appear and continue cooking until golden brown.

Breakfast Rice

Cook rice as directed on package. Brown rice offers more nutrients and has a nutty taste that children like. Grind brown rice in the blender before cooking. This will make it easier for small children to chew. Then try adding raisins, dry chopped fruit, peach slices, apple chunks, or chopped celery to the rice while it is steaming. Sprinkle a little cinnamon on each serving. If a sweeter rice is desired, drizzle a little honey or molasses on to taste.

Butterfly in my Breakfast
(serves 2)

2 canned pineapple rings
½ apple (cut into 2 wedges)
4 small carrot sticks
2 pieces of whole wheat toast

Cut pineapple rings in half. Place 1 apple wedge, cut side down, in the center of each piece of toast. Lay the cut piece of pineapple rings on each side of apple to form butterfly wings. Add 2 carrot sticks to each butterfly to make the antennae. Serve with milk for a complete breakfast.

Dolly Delight
(serves 2)

2 canned apricot halves
½ cup cottage cheese
¼ cup grated cheddar cheese
4 small raisins
4 small carrot sticks
4 pieces of melba toast

Put 1/4 cup cottage cheese (drop by ice-cream scoop) in the center of each plate. Place 1 apricot half on each plate next to cottage cheese. This will be the doll's head. Use raisins for the eyes, the grated cheese for hair and the carrot sticks for arms. Place 2 melba toast at the bottom of each doll for shoes. Serve immediately.

Baked Apples

apples
cinnamon
honey or molasses and butter (if desired)

Core but do not peel each apple. Place each apple in a baking dish. If apple will not stand upright, slice some off the bottom to make a flat surface. Drizzle honey or molasses inside of apple. Sprinkle with cinnamon and dot with butter if desired. Cover dish with aluminum foil. Bake 15–20 minutes at 350 degrees.

Apples and Muffin
(serves 2)

1 apple
2 English muffins, split
Cinnamon

Core, peel, and slice apple into rings. Separate each English muffin into halves. Lightly butter each half of muffin. Place apple rings on top of each muffin. Sprinkle with cinnamon. Put on rack under broiler until apples are tender and brown. Serve warm.

Morning Almost-Popovers

1 cup milk
1 cup whole wheat flour + 1/2 tsp. salt
1 tbsp. oil
¼ tsp. vanilla
2 eggs

Mix milk, flour, oil and salt together. Add vanilla and stir in eggs one at a time. Beat until smooth. Fill greased and floured muffin pans ¾ full and bake at 425 degrees for 15 minutes. Reduce temperature to 350 degrees and bake another 15 to 20 minutes.

Easy Granola

¼ cup honey
½ cup water
½ cup vegetable oil
2 tsp. pure vanilla
1 tsp. cinnamon

Combine all ingredients and heat until the mixture just begins to boil. Then quickly stir in the following ingredients:

7 cups rolled oats
½ cup sunflower seeds
½ cup flaked coconut
¼ cup wheat germ

Spread on large cookie sheet and bake in a preheated oven at 250 degrees. Stir mixture often so it will not burn. Cook until a rich brown. This takes approximately 45 minutes. Remove from oven and cool. Add raisins or dried fruit for added flavor. Serve as a cereal with milk or by itself for a snack.

Snacks

Should day-care children be given daily snacks? In a word—YES! Small children need food at regular intervals to maintain their energy. Actually, day-care children should have a mid-morning and a mid-afternoon snack. This is required if you are in the U.S.D.A. food program.

Snacks should be both appetizing and nutritious. Children will want to snack on the same foods you do, so set a good example. You can make appealing snacks from foods you have on hand.

Beverages may be served in the form of milk, water, fruit juices, fruit popsicles, fruit shakes, and vegetable juices. All are guaranteed to hit the spot.

For something to go with the beverage, try vegetable sticks with cottage cheese dips, cheese logs, apple wedges with peanut butter, soft pretzels, muffins, or banana bread. If the children are extra hungry, try melting cheese on toast. Try some of the ideas and recipes that follow, and have fun varying combinations.

Quick Snacks

All of the following quick snacks are easy to prepare.

1. raisin toast
   milk
2. bagel
   grapes
3. toast
   orange wedges
4. bran muffin
   applejuice
5. oatmeal cookies
   milk
6. baked apples
   wheat crackers
7. rice cakes with
   melted grated cheese
8. pancake or
   peanut butter sandwich
   milk
9. fruit plate
   soda crackers
10. banana slices
    milk
11. frozen grapes
    Rye Krisp
12. watermelon balls
    toasted English muffin
13. kiwi and banana slices
    rice cakes
14. hot rice with molasses
    milk

15. applesauce
    toast
16. tortillas
    fruit cocktail
17. graham crackers
    milk
18. granola
    apple juice
19. celery
    peanut butter
20. saltine crackers
    cheese slices
21. frozen blueberries
    milk
22. biscuits
    pear sauce
23. cottage cheese
    peach slices
24. hard boiled egg
    orange juice
25. apricots
    cornbread
26. sliced carrots
    and turnips
    cottage cheese dip
27. strawberry shake
    wheatsworth crackers
28. cottage cheese
    on toast
29. cucumber spears
    French bread with butter
30. melba toast
    cherries
31. Purple Cow
    peanut butter cookies
32. soda crackers
    pineapple chunks

FUN WITH SNACKS

Beverages

Strawberry Shake

¾ cup milk
5 frozen strawberries
1 tsp. vanilla

Blend until smooth and frothy. Serve immediately.

Purple Cow

¼ cup grape juice
½ cup milk
½ banana

Blend until smooth and serve.

Orange Julius

½ cup milk per child
1 egg for every 2 children
½ cup orange juice per child
2 tbsp. honey
4 ice cubes

Blend until smooth. Chill well and mix again just before serving.

Apple-Pineapple Cooler

1 cup unsweetened apple juice
⅔ cup unsweetened pineapple juice
⅓ cup orange juice
2 tsp. lemon juice (freshly squeezed)

Combine all ingredients; chill and serve.

Raspberry-Fruit Drink

¼ cup frozen raspberries
1 cup pineapple-grapefruit juice
lemon wedges

Blend raspberries and juice until smooth; garnish with lemon and serve.

Tropical Twist

1 cup unsweetened pineapple juice
1 ripe banana
1 tsp. honey
1 tbsp. lime juice
2 ice cubes

Blend all ingredients until frothy and serve.

Breads, Muffins, Bars, and Treats

Banana Bread

    1¾ cup unsifted flour
    1 tbsp. baking powder
    ½ tsp. salt

Mix thoroughly; set aside.

    ¾ cup sugar
    ½ cup shortening
    2 eggs
    1 tbsp. cinnamon
    2 cups mashed bananas

Mix together until light and fluffy. Mix in the bananas. Add dry ingredients; stir until smooth. Pour into greased 9 × 5 inch pain and bake at 350 degrees for 50 to 60 minutes. Bread will be firm to the touch. Cool on rack for 10 minutes and remove from the pan. Slice and serve.

Granola Balls

    ¼ cup old-fashioned peanut butter
    ¼ cup honey

        Heat ingredients until lukewarm. Mix well.

    2 cups granola
    ½ tsp. wheat germ

Stir into heated mixture. Mix well and scoop out balls with small scoop. Roll in sesame seeds.

Date Nut Muffins

2 tbsp. margarine, melted
½ cup buttermilk
1 egg

Beat egg. Add margarine and buttermilk.

1 cup flour
1½ tsp. baking powder
⅛ tsp. salt
¼ tsp soda
¼ cup chopped walnuts
½ cup finely chopped dates
1 tsp. cinnamon

Mix all ingredients together. Add to egg mixture and stir to blend. Bake in greased muffin tins at 350 degrees for 20 minutes. Serve warm.

Granola Bars

2 eggs

Beat eggs well.

2 cups granola
½ cup coconut

Stir into beaten eggs. Pour into a greased 9 inch square pan. Bake 20 minutes at 350 degrees. Cut into bars. Frost with 1 cup peanut butter mixed with 2 tbsp. honey. Garnish with coconut.

Peanut Butter Nuggets

1 cup peanut butter
1 tsp. lemon juice
¼ tsp. salt

Mix together.

    1 can condensed milk
    1 cup chopped raisins

Gradually stir in milk. Add raisins. Drop by teaspoon onto greased cookie sheet. Bake 10 minutes at 375 degrees. Makes 36.

Cranberry Quick Bread

    1¾ cups flour
    1 tbsp. baking powder
    ¾ tsp. salt
    1 tsp. cinnamon

Sift all ingredients together. Set aside.

    1 egg, slightly beaten
    ½ cup honey
    1 tbsp. grated orange peel
    ¾ cup milk
    2 tbsp. melted butter

Combine ingredients. Pour all at once into dry ingredients. Mix just until moistened. Stir in 1 cup raw cranberries. Pour into greased loaf pan. Bake at 325 degrees for 1 hour.

Homemade Jell-O

    ½ package unflavored gelatin
    ½ cup 100% fruit juice

Soak gelatin in juice for 5 minutes. Heat until the gelatin dissolves.

    ½ cup 100% fruit juice
    Juice from half a lemon

Add to gelatin mixture and stir well. Cool slightly. Add any sliced fruit and chill until set.

Peanut Butter Play Dough

1 cup peanut butter
3 tbsp. honey
Nonfat dry milk

Mix peanut butter and honey. Add enough dry milk until mixture is of a stiff consistency. Shape and eat.

Potato Puffs

½ cup mashed potatoes
1 cup dry milk
½ tsp. vanilla
2 tbsp. honey
sesame seeds, almonds

Mix potatoes, dry milk, vanilla, and honey together. Add more dry milk if necessary to make stiff balls. Make small balls, roll in sesame seeds, press an almond on top. Bake at 350 degrees for 15 minutes until golden brown.

Juice-Sicles

1 quart 100% juice (orange, grape, pinappple, etc.)

Pour into small 5-oz. paper cups. Freeze for ½ hour and then put plastic spoons into center of cups to use for holder. Return to freezer. Freeze until solid. Warm outside of cup with your hand, invert, and remove from cup. Enjoy!

Fruit and Cheese Kabobs

Cut fruit into small pieces and alternate with small cheese cubes. Spear onto strong toothpicks. Serve.

Refried Bean Dip

Heat together one can of refried beans, add enough milk to soften to dip consistency. Serve with fresh vegetable sticks.

Frozen Bananas

Peel bananas, dip in lemon juice, roll in coconut, chopped nuts, or fine granola. Insert wooden skewers halfway into each. Freeze until firm.

Tofu Strawberry Pudding

10½ oz. tofu
1¼ cups chopped strawberries
½ banana
1 tsp. vanilla
2 tbsp. honey

Puree all ingredients and serve chilled.

Freezer Finger Goodies

Freeze any of the following. Serve frozen treats anytime for snack.

seedless grapes	banana slices
peas	orange sections
blueberries	watermelon balls
raspberries	canteloupe balls
marion berries	kiwi slices

Instant Sandwiches

Mix peanut butter with any of the following:

molasses	grated apples
apple sauce	bananas

grated carrots
chopped dates

raisins
grated cabbage

Serve on any of the following:

graham crackers
rice cakes
biscuits
celery
tortillas

apple slices
rye crisp
pancakes
muffins
soda crackers

Lunch/Dinner

The lunch meal offers the best opportunity to enjoy your day care children. After an active morning, it is a welcome break in the day. Children should have a quiet time just before lunch. Play music, read a story, or just have them rest for a few minutes, before they wash their hands to eat. This will calm them down and set a social and relaxed mood for mealtime.

This is a time to encourage socialization in the form of pleasant conversation between the children and yourself. Allow for different eating patterns and allow children to participate in the entire mealtime process. Children can help prepare certain foods. They can scoop, measure, mix, stir, press appropriate button on blender, oil and flour baking tins. They will pick out words or letters on food packages. They can wash up before eating, set the table, and clear their own spot after the meal is finished. Even a toddler will enjoy being put in charge of the napkin detail. The napkins may be dropped several times, but the toddler will thoroughly enjoy making this important contribution. By allowing small children to do even the simplest task, you will be helping them to develop small-motor coordination and self-confidence. Some spillage is bound to happen. Small-scale assignments will avert major mess or waste.

During the meal encourage your day-care children to try one bite of everything. Set a good example for them by keeping your dislikes to yourself. Children learn food likes and dislikes through imitation. If they see you look with distaste at peas, for example, they will pick up your dislike. Introduce new foods occasionally. Serve a favorite food with the new one. This will help them to associate their liking of the favorite food with the taste of the new food. New foods that are served in a special way can often encourage children to try them. So experiment, and have fun in preparing the lunch meal.

Remember though, to never force a child to eat. Do not use food as a punishment or a reward. Avoid the old cliché, "Children are starving, and you leave food on your plate." This only leads to food problems later in life. Children sometimes find it hard to clean their plates of every speck of food. Encourage them to eat as much as they feel like, and that is all. Keep the mealtime atmosphere unhurried and happy, so that the meal can be enjoyed to the fullest. This is a good time to reenforce acceptable table manners. Teach the children how to use a fork, knife, or spoon, as well as when to use each one. Show them how a napkin rests on a lap; how to ask someone to pass the milk; the proper way to drink; the value of wiping their chins. A few extra minutes on your part can save embarrassment on the child's part. Children who learn good table manners feel better about themselves. And about you.

Lunch Tips

1. Grill tuna sandwiches for a different taste.
2. Serve children on small plates instead of large.
3. Put chicken salad into ice-cream cones for small hands.
4. Plan bright, colorful food combinations.
5. Use less spices or condiments in children's food.
6. Serve fruit cocktail in hollowed-out orange shells.
7. Prepare raw vegetables and fruits as finger food.
8. Steam vegetables to maintain flavor.
9. Cut sandwiches into interesting shapes.
10. Have an indoor picnic if it is raining.
11. Keep a jar of sprouts growing to add to sandwiches and salads.
12. Try whole wheat or vegetable pastas.
13. Make it yourself whenever possible. It will save you money, and taste better. The children will love helping you.

14. Cook without salt. Season with garlic and herbs.
15. Serve fresh fruit for desserts rather than white sugar products.
16. Use less red meat. Use more fish, poultry, and beans for protein.
17. Use whole wheat flours when possible.

Fun with Lunch/Dinner

Chicken Salad

2 cups cooked, cubed chicken
1 cup chopped celery
½ cup apple chunks or seedless grapes
¼ tsp. salt
¼ tsp. chopped dill
¼ cup mayonnaise

Mix all ingredients together. Serve in lettuce cups.

3-Bean Salad

1 can kidney beans
1 can garbanzo beans
1 can green or yellow wax beans
¼ cup chopped onions
2 tbsp. honey
½ cup Italian dressing

Combine all ingredients. Allow to chill for 2 to 4 hours.

Easy Fruit Salad

1 can pineapple chunks
2 sliced bananas
1 cup apple chunks

2 tbsp. honey
¼ cup lemon juice

Combine all ingredients. Serve immediately.

Easy Chili
(serves 4)

Brown ½ pound ground beef in a skillet. Drain fat off. Pour in 2 cans kidney beans, ½ cup chopped celery and ¼ cup chopped onions. If you want more of a chili flavor, add 1 tbsp. chili powder. Simmer until celery is tender. Serve over hot rice.

Vegetable Macaroni
(serves 4)

Cook 8 oz. of macaroni until done, drain and set aside. Whirl in the blender:

1½ cups diced cheddar cheese
1½ cups milk
1½ tbsp. flour
1 tsp. salt
1 tbsp. butter

Blend well. Mix drained macaroni with any leftover vegetables (corn, peas, green beans, etc.). Put the macaroni and vegetables into baking dish. Pour liquid mixture over the top and stir. Dot top with pieces of cheddar cheese. Bake at 350 degrees until cheese is melted and mixture is bubbly.

Tostados
(serves 4)

1 can refried beans
8 corn tortillas
1 cup grated Monterey Jack cheese

2 cups shredded lettuce
2 tomatoes, chopped

Heat refried beans until they bubble slightly. Stir often to prevent scorching. Warm tortillas by frying them in a skillet with a little oil. Drain tortillas on paper towels. Place one tortilla on each plate. Spread warm refried beans on each one. Add grated cheese. Top with lettuce and tomatoes. Serve with mild taco sauce.

Taco Salad
(serves 4–6)

1 lb ground beef
½ cup chopped celery

Brown both in skillet. In a large bowl, add:

1 cup grated cheese
4 cups shredded lettuce
1 cup chopped tomatoes
1 cup broken tortilla chips

Mix in warm ground beef. Add ½ cup French dressing. Stir and serve warm.

French-Style Dressing

1 cup tomato juice
2 tbsp. lemon juice
½ tsp. oregano
¼ tsp. garlic powder
pinch of pepper

Put all ingredients in a jar and shake well. Store in a covered jar in the refrigerator.

Vegetable Soup
(serves 6)

4 cups chicken or beef stock
¼ tsp. garlic powder
pinch of pepper
1 onion, chopped
1 cup chopped celery
4 carrots, sliced into thin rounds
½ cabbage, shredded
1 cup canned tomatoes

Bring stock to a boil. Add garlic, pepper, onion, celery, and carrots. Simmer until vegetables are tender. Add cabbage and tomatoes. Simmer until cabbage is cooked. Serve.

Baked Mini Meat Loaves
(serves 4)

¾ pound lean ground beef
¾ cup uncooked oatmeal
¼ onion, grated
¼ tsp. salt
⅛ tsp. pepper

Mix all ingredients together. Form into four loaves about 2 inches high. Place in a large ungreased baking pan. Bake at 375 degrees until brown and cooked through, about 25 minutes. Drain off fat before serving.

Baked Cod and Peas
(serves 4)

1 pound cod
1 10 oz. package frozen green peas
¼ cup lemon juice
1 tbsp. butter

½ tsp. garlic powder
½ tsp. basil

Put cod on large piece of aluminum foil. Pour frozen peas on top of cod. Melt butter and add lemon juice, garlic powder and basil. Pour butter mixture over fish and peas. Seal foil tightly. Bake in preheated oven at 350 degrees for 20 to 25 minutes. Serve immediately.

Zucchini Layered Casserole

2 cups zucchini, thinly sliced with skin
1 10 oz. package frozen corn, thawed
1 10 oz. package frozen spinach, thawed
1 cup grated Monterey Jack cheese
½ cup chopped onion
1 cup tomato sauce

Spread 1 cup of zucchini in bottom of greased 9 × 13 pan. Spread corn on top of zucchini and follow with spinach. Spread ½ cup grated cheese and chopped onion over spinach. Pour on ½ cup of tomato sauce. Add remaining 1 cup of zucchini and top with remaining ½ cup tomato sauce. Spread cheese on top. ke 30–40 minutes at 350 degrees. For a moister casserole cover with aluminum foil the first 20 minutes of cooking. Casserole is done when the zucchini is tender.

Chapter 5

TOYS THAT TEACH FUN

The use of toys in the day-care situation can be both fun and educational. Through their use, children develop both the mind and the body. But choosing the right toys can be confusing, especially with the wide selection that is available.

Asking yourself these three questions when purchasing a toy for your day-care children will help you choose.

1. Is it suitable for the age of the child?
2. Is it versatile? Can it be used in more than one way?
3. Is it safe and durable?

If you can answer yes to each of these questions, then the toy you've selected should provide hours of enjoyment. Reconsider your purchase if you answer no to any of the questions.

Remember that as a day-care provider, it is your responsibility to make sure the toys used are safe. Small Leggos may be ideal for a four-year-old; but could be swallowed by an infant. Anything that a baby can put into his mouth, he will. So, read all manufacturers' cautions and recommendations that are provided for each toy.

To aid you in your selection, a list of recommended toys follows, arranged by children's ages. Naturally, you will want to add your own ideas. This is not an entire list of possibilities. It has been designed to use as a guide.

Some toys have been starred. These can be easily made at home. Following the list are directions to make each such toy.

Draw on your own creativity to make toys. For further ideas, think back to the toys you made as a child. Ask your day-care children to help. They will probably give you many new ideas for usable toys.

Toys can be readily purchased at lawn sales, rummage sales, and thrift shops. Just be sure to examine each toy carefully first. Is it missing parts? Is it broken? Has the paint been chipped, so as to cut small fingers? Will it last? Asking yourself a few questions can prevent your throwing away money on a toy you'll later throw away.

Shop carefully and you will enjoy the toys yourself, and the children will pick up on your own enthusiasm.

TOYS FOR EACH AGE

Infancy to Six Months

> stuffed animal (small)
> soft ball (large)
> colorful pictures
> mobile*
> soft plastic doll
> teething ring/beads
> soft blocks
> rattle
> cradle bells*
> musical toys

Six to Twelve Months

> soft hairbrush
> soft blocks

rubber hammer
plastic serving spoons
cloth books*
rubber bath toys
rolling ball with vinyl window
teething toys
rag doll
squeeze toys

One Year

hand puppets
push toys
picture books
colorful ball
play trucks
drum*
pyramid rings
small ride-on bike
toy telephone

Eighteen Months

wooden cars
colorful wood blocks
Duplo building toys
sandbox*
bucket and shovel
pull toys
cobbler's bench
plastic hats (fireman, cowboy, Robin Hood, spaceman)
plastic bowls, cups, spoons
ride-on toys
metal coffee pot with Tupperware containers
balloons
fingerpaints

Two Years

- magnetic letter board
- chalkboard
- story books
- building blocks
- rocking horse
- coloring books
- crayons
- play table and chairs
- simple puzzles
- small boxes
- Peg-Board*
- Hungry Hippo game
- cards
- waffle balls
- small plastic animals
- magnetic shapes*
- empty clean food boxes
- play dough*
- tricycle
- beanbags
- bubble-blowing set
- top
- dress-up clothes
- handbag
- speak and say games
- chalkboard*

Three Years

- paper
- pencils
- stapler
- jigsaws

letter blocks
toy airplane
Weebles
playhouse*
tent
xylophone
masks
circus animals
small cards
small dolls
doll clothes
threading cards
plastic garden tools
fat plastic bat
number and letter books
hats
soccer ball

Four Years

simple card game
painting book
watercolors
play clock*
hospital kit
play money
clay
tents
sewing cards
threading beads
Nerf football
Nerf basketball
baskets
preschool record player

records
toy microphone
plastic bowls
Simon Says game
stickers*

Five Years

easy-to-read stories
dominos
cards
board games
roller skates
jump rope
yo-yo
toy typewriter
stilts*
toy recorder
jacks
kite
word games
frisbee

TOYS TO MAKE

1. Mobile
   Use frame from an old mobile. Attach a string and hang anything light and colorful: silk flower, balloon, plastic spoon, plastic bell, plastic rings.
   Babies especially enjoy the primary colors—bright reds, yellows, and blues. When arranging your mobile, display the objects at different lengths. Allow it to stay up only a few days. Then replace it with another creation.
2. Cradle Bells
   Measure the width of the crib. Cut or buy a ¼" dowel the

width of the crib plus 4 inches. Starting at one end of the dowel, cricle it with 2"-wide silk ribbon. When the dowel is covered, glue the ends, and allow to dry. Now take six 3"-round bells and tie 6"-lengths of ribbon (in various bright colors and lengths) to each bell. Then tie ribbon and bells onto the dowel. Tie ends of dowel to each side of crib.

3. Cloth Book

You will need:

    8 pieces of heavy broadcloth in bright colors (6" × 4")
    thread
    needle
    pinking shears
    liquid embroidery

Pink the edges of each piece of fabric. Draw a picture with the liquid embroidery on each piece: a ball, a tree, a doll, a car, a bear. Now stack the fabric so that book is 6" long and 4" wide. Sew together to form book.

Variation: Sew buttons on one page, a zipper on another. Use rickrack to form design. Keep it colorful!

4. Drum

Simply put the plastic lid on an empty coffee can. Tape it on securely. Give the child a plastic spoon and your drum is completed.

Variation: Use an oatmeal container. Be sure to tape the top on.

5. Sandbox

Indoors: Fill a small inflatable swimming pool full of oatmeal. It's fun to play in and easy to vacuum up when done.

Outdoors: Fill an old plastic children's pool or an old plastic baby bathtub with sand. You can purchase fine sand at your local home improvement store or at a rock quarry. Minimal expense for hours of fun.

6. Peg-Board

You will need:

    2 pieces of Masonite Peg-Board
    sandpaper
    golf tees

Cut two pieces of Masonite Peg-Board to desired size and shape. Sand all edges well. Glue one piece of Masonite Peg-Board on top of the other. Make sure the holes are lined up properly. Sand sharp ends of golf tees to make them smooth and blunt. Paint, if desired.

7. Magnetic Shapes

You will need:

scraps of felt
old greeting cards
roll of peel-and-stick magnet tape
scissors or pinking shears
fabric glue
glitter

Cut various shapes from the felt: pear, orange half, apple, triangle, ball, square, tree.

Draw and cut out designs, apply glue and glitter. Allow to dry completely. Attach a 2" strip of magnet to the back of the shape.

Variation: Cut pictures out of old greeting cards: flowers, baskets, animals. Then follow directions above.

8. Play Dough

Mix one cup of flour and ½ cup of salt. Add one tbsp. of cooking oil and two tbsp. of water. Add water as needed to make the dough pliable. Knead well.

Mix in a few drops of food coloring if desired. This dough is edible but not tasty. Keep it in a sealed plastic bag in the refrigerator. It should keep for weeks of use.

9. Chalkboard

You will need:

chalkboard paint
plywood
molding
chalk
erasers
sandpaper

Cut plywood to desired size and shape. Sand surface and edges until smooth. Paint surface with chalkboard paint, allow to dry completely. Attach molding to bottom for a dust tray. If attaching a large chalkboard to a plaster wall, use molly screws to hold in position.

10. Jigsaw

Have the children color a favorite picture. Cover it front and back with peel-and-stick clear plastic. Then simply cut into the desired number of pieces.

11. Playhouse

Get a large appliance box from a local store. Cut doors and windows. Let the children color it. Set it in a corner for them to play in.

12. Play Clock

You will need:

 2 paper plates
 felt pens (various colors)
 paper fastener

Color and number one paper plate to resemble a clock. Cut two arrows, one long and one short, from the other paper plate. Attach the arrows to the center of your play clock with the paper fastener. Keep the clock hands loose enough to move them around the face of the clock to point to different times.

13. Stickers

You will need:

 several sheets of canning or peel-and-stick labels
 paper
 colored pencils

Simply decorate each label with any patterns you like: sun, rainbow, stars, animals, flowers, names, or sayings; or symbols of a current holiday (hearts, bunny, flag, jack-o-lantern, turkey, wreath).

14. Stilts

You will need:

2 4" pieces of PCV plastic pipe (48" in length)
2 2" × 4" × 4" pieces of pine
4 ¾" × 7" carriage bolts
4 ¾" washers and nuts

Drill one ¾ hole through 4" × 48" PCV pipe 6" from one end. Drill a second ¾" hole 8" from end. Repeat on next PCV pipe. Make sure carriage bolts slide through easily.

Now mark the two holes on the two 2" × 4" × 4" pieces of pine. Drill holes in pine. Attach pine blocks to PCU pipe with carriage bolts, washers, and nuts.

Demonstrate safe use of stilts to children. Stand back and enjoy watching the children have fun with their new toy.

OUTSIDE PLAY AREAS

"Can we go outside now?" That question is heard more times by day-care providers than any other. Children, it seems, do not care whether the sun is brightly shining, or it is pouring rain. The question is the same.

Day-care providers recognize that it is natural for children to run, jump, and climb. These are necessary activities if children are to develop coordination, creativity, and self-assurance. Outdoor play offers scope for all this.

First, children learn through experience. In a well organized outside play area, children have the opportunity to use many muscle groups that they do not use indoors. By developing their muscles, they learn to control them. A toddler who is learning to walk at first falls more than he stands. After a while, though, he begins controlling his leg muscles, and is soon walking without falling.

It is through this muscle control that coordination is developed. To children, running, jumping, and climbing are ways to have fun. They do not realize the benefits their bodies receive from such activities. Table 5-1, from the Portland, Oregon Public Schools Guide to Playground Equipment, lists the basic motor components: strength, endurance, agility, flexibility, coordi-

Playground Equipment and Developmental Activities

Equipment Item	Strength Shoulder	Arm	Abdominal	Back	Legs	Endurance Cardio-Respiratory	Muscular	Agility	Flexibility	Coordination	Symmetry	Balance	Body Awareness in space
FIXED EQUIPMENT													
1. Balance Beams													
a. level	★	★	✓	✓	✓			★	★				
b. inclined	★	★	✓	✓	✓			★	★				
2. Bridges													
a. ramp	✓	✓	★	✓	✓		★	✓		✓	✓	✓	
b. rigid					✓							✓	
c. arch				✓	✓	✓	✓					✓	✓
3. Cargo Nets and Rope Climb													
a. lean-to	✓	✓	✓	✓	✓		✓	✓	✓	✓	✓		
b. tepee	✓	✓	✓	✓	✓		✓	✓	✓	✓	✓		
c. rope climb	✓	✓	✓	✓	✓	✓	✓	✓		✓			✓

4. Domes and Ladders														
a. geodesic	✓	✓	✓	✓	✓	✓	✓	✓	✓	✓	✓	✓	✓	✓
b. archway climber	✓	✓	✓	✓	✓	✓	✓	✓	✓	✓		✓	✓	✓
c. tire trees	✓	✓	✓		✓	✓	✓	✓	✓		✓		✓	✓
d. horizontal ladder	✓	✓	✓	✓	✓	✓	✓	✓	✓		✓		✓	✓
5. Bars														
a. horizontal bar	✓	✓	✓		★	✓	✓	★	★		✓		✓	✓
6. Platforms			✓											
7. Slides														
a. platform		✓		✓							✓		✓	✓
b. fire pole	✓	✓	✓	★	✓						✓			
c. ladder slide	✓	✓			✓		✓	✓	✓		✓		✓	✓
8. Progressive logs														
a. round logs			✓	✓	✓	✓	✓	✓	✓				✓	✓
b. square logs			✓	✓	✓	✓	✓	✓	✓				✓	✓
9. Tires														
a. Caterpillar tires		✓	✓	✓									✓	✓
b. obstacle tires			✓	✓			✓				✓		✓	✓

117

Playground Equipment and Developmental Activities (continued)

	Basic Motor Components											
	Strength					Endurance		Agility	Flexibility	Coordination	Symmetry	Balance	Body Awareness in space
Equipment Item	Shoulder	Arm	Abdominal	Back	Legs	Cardio-Respiratory	Muscular						
FIXED EQUIPMENT													
MOVING EQUIPMENT													
1. Moving Balance Beam	★	★	★	★	★			✔		✔		✔	✔
2. Clatter Bridge	★	★	★	★	★			✔		✔		✔	✔
3. Log Roll	✔	✔	✔	✔	✔	✔	✔	✔		✔	✔		
4. Spring Platform	★	★	✔	✔	✔	✔	✔	✔		✔	✔	✔	✔
5. Tire Swing	✔	✔	✔	✔	★					✔		✔	✔
6. Tire Raft	✔	✔					✔			✔		✔	✔

✔ = PRIMARY VALUE   ★ = SECONDARY VALUE

Revised 3/80

nation, symmetry, balance, and body awareness. The Table then evaluates standard playground equipment as to primary and secondary value. Notice that there are only two pieces of equipment that offer primary value in all areas: the geodesic dome and the archway climber.

This does not mean that you cannot have an outside play area without these. On the contrary, this only shows the need for children to exercise all upper and lower muscle groups to develop coordination. Include something to climb in your play area, if you possibly can. Even a rope tied securely from a tree or patio beam will offer hours of fun. Make sure you use a strong rope, tie knots in it, and clear away obstacles within swinging range.

Second is creativity. How do you enable children to be creative in an outside play area? Space is the key. Allow enough space for building, digging, filling, and even destroying. Children can be very creative with very little. A large tire filled with sand can become a hub of activity. There, children can build roads or sand castles. They can dig holes and refill them again. Try to provide an assortment of inexpensive implements (cans, scoops, shovels, bowls, spoons, strainers). These will give children hours of fun. Remember to cover the sand when not in use. This will protect it from the neighborhood cats.

Water is another source in which to encourage creativity. Fill an old baby bathtub with water. The children will float, sink, and drop their toys in the water to watch the results. Supply a wide variety of plastic bottles, watering cans, boats, bath toys, cups, spoons, corks. For added fun, try putting in a few drops of food coloring. The colored water will open up many new ideas. Children will use their imagination to create games. You can even give them pails of water and old paint brushes to paint the sidewalk on a hot afternoon. Or, allow would-be painters to paint the house. Both the sidewalk and the house will return to their original color when the water evaporates. Water play will always encourage creativity in children.

If water is available for play, the children will not care whether they are playing outdoors or indoors. When the weather is not suitable for playing outdoors, fill the sink with colored water. Lay towels on the floor to soak up the overflow. Provide various measuring cups, and help your day-care children learn what the various measures are. Soon, they will be able to distinguish one cup from one-fourth of a cup, and one teaspoon from one tablespoon. Or, they may make their own methods of measuring.

Each child is creative in his own way. If you asked five small children to draw a happy face, you would receive five variations. It is important to encourage this creativity. At times it may be hard to understand exactly how the disassembling of a toy, or the splashing of water, can in any way encourage creativity. But trying new ways to redirect the flow of water over the counters is an expression of creativity through which children learn.

When you are organizing your outside play area, plan to include materials that will stimulate your children's creativity. Large trucks with compartments for transporting goods, for example, are far superior to trucks with fancy painting. Any play item you select that will excite curiosity, will encourage all your day-care children to be creative.

Self-assurance is just as important as coordination and creativity to your children. If they are to develop a strong sense of who they are, they must develop self-assurance. How can you help them to do this?

As a day-care provider you can help your children to develop self-assurance by allowing them to conquer obstacles. Take, for example, children's attitude toward the various climbing structures. Their first approach is a very cautious one. They may at first climb only one rung, and then get down. The next time, they will climb two rungs. This will continue until the children gain confidence. Then, they will climb to the top over and over again. They have now gained self-assurance by conquering an obstacle.

When you allow them the freedom to create their own obstacles, you will see their self-assurance grow. Children will demonstrate this newfound self-assurance by creating their own climbing structures. They will push boxes, chairs, or stools together, and then climb with extreme confidence. Have you ever noticed a child's face sparkle when he has walked a balance beam, or climbed a tree, for the first time? Initially, his face reflects his determination to accomplish the task; but watch that same face change when the task is conquered! It will now reflect a sense of worth, joy, and confidence. That self-assurance will be carried on to conquer future obstacles.

You might ask who can afford to install an expensive outside play area. It is a fact that day-care providers are usually extremely limited in their financial resources. But with a little ingenuity, research, and effort you can provide an exciting play area at a relatively low cost.

The first thing to do is to make a list of all your possible resources. Take your finances into account. How much can you spend on a play area? Take into consideration your existing play equipment, the size of your proposed play area, and the amount of time you can give to the project. This is an important first step. It will provide you with an overview of the situation. You may be surprised at the quantity of your resources when they are written down.

Next, look through self-help books for ideas. You can borrow several from your local library. Write down any item that will suit your needs, and can easily be constructed. The only prerequisite to keep in mind when reviewing these books is safety. Make sure that each item can be anchored to the ground to prevent possible mishaps.

After you have a list of possible playground equipment, make a parts list. Include every nut and bolt. This will help you to be able to estimate the cost. Take your list to your local hardware or lumber store. Talk to the salesperson about what you are trying to do and ask for suggestions. Such stores may have free information pamphlets that are of help. When all information has been gathered, you will be able to choose specific equipment to build. Doing it yourself can be fun, if you plan in advance.

If you do not have the money, talent, or time to devote to constructing your outside play area, you might look for freebies. Sometimes you will find old swing sets at low cost in the ads of your local newspaper. Then the only problem will be getting it to your home.

Toys from tires

Another inexpensive idea is to use old tires. You could ask your local tire store for used bias ply tires. They probably will give them to you free or for a small fee. Make sure that they are not steel or glass belted tires, but are bias ply only. Ask your tire dealer to show you the difference. When steel or glass is exposed, children can get cut or scraped on the exposed edges.

You will find many uses for old tires in various sizes. Some ideas are offered here. If the proposed design does not suit your needs, change it to meet your specifications. Always make it safe by anchoring the structure to the ground. When using tires, it is a good idea to drill drainage holes in each tire. Water can collect in them, making a breeding ground for mosquitoes and other bugs. There have also been cases of accidental drownings in the 6-foot and larger-size tire.

Caterpillar Tires

Safety Considerations

1. Connecting hardware should not be sharp.
2. Anchor bottom portion of tire.
3. Seal off opening of first and last tire.
4. Use 6- or 8-ply bias tires.

Inspection Considerations

1. Check for loose tires.
2. Check for exposed metal in tires.

Benefits

1. Balance and coordination are developed.
2. Uneven surface helps to develop eye/foot coordination.

Climbing Tires

Safety Considerations

1. Can use large 4- to 6-ft. tires.
2. Bury at least ⅓ of tire in ground if in standing position.

Inspection Considerations

1. Check tire for wear and exposed metal wire.
2. Check that tire is secure in position.

Instruction to Children

   No pushing or shoving off tire.

Benefit

   Develops balance and coordination.

Obstacle Tires

Safety Considerations

1. Use auto-size 6-ply bias tires.
2. Firmly connect tires to each other.
3. Secure to the ground.

Inspection Considerations

1. Check monthly to see if tires are loose.
2. Check for exposed metal within the tires.

Instructions to Children

1. No pushing.
2. One child at a time.

Benefits

1. Develops eye/foot coordination.
2. Strengthens calf and thigh muscles.

Tire Swing

Safety Considerations

1. Maximum height, 7 ft.

2. Auto tire only.
3. 6-ply bias tire.
4. Use heavy-weight rope.

Inspection Considerations

1. Check to make sure rope is secure.
2. Check tire for wear.

Instructions to Children

1. Only one child on swing at a time.
2. No toys in swing area.

Benefits

1. Upper arms are somewhat strengthened.
2. Eye/hand/foot coordination.

Tire Tree

Safety Considerations

1. Maximum height, 7 ft.
2. Group tires close together on post.
3. Anchor with a carriage bolt, nut, and washer.
4. 6- or 8-ply tires (bias).
5. Auto or pickup tires.

Inspection Considerations

1. Check for loose tires.
2. Check for wood rot.

Instructions to Children

1. No jumping from tires.
2. Don't step on others' fingers or hands.

Benefits

1. Balancing.
2. Eye/hand coordination.
3. Upper arm, calfs, and thighs are strengthened.

Other Toys

Boards in all sizes can add another exciting dimension to your outside play area. They can be used for climbing, jumping, sliding, balancing, and even teetering. Children will use them to create bridges, tables, boats, forts, houses, racetracks, barricades.

Choose sturdy weathered or new boards of varying lengths and widths. Boards that are either 2" × 4" or 1" × 10" in size are especially useful. It is a good idea to finish the boards, so that they will not warp or splinter if left outside.

Attach cleats to both ends of the boards; then the boards will not slip off whatever they are propped against. This is done simply by cutting a 2" × 2" strip of wood the width of the board and attaching it with screws. If the board is to be used for climbing, space the cleats 8 to 10 inches apart.

Teach your day-care children how to carry boards properly, and how to check each one for safety. For instance, the cleat should be in position so as not to let the board slip. Some ideas for use are:

1. To construct a balance beam, lay a 1" × 10" × 8" board on the ground. Place one old tire under each end of the board so that the cleats are on the outside of each tire.
2. To make a ladder use a board that has cleats spaced every 8 to 10 inches on the front. Make sure it has two cleats on the back to prevent slipping. Simply prop it against a tree, jungle gym, or climbing box.
3. To make a teeter-totter lay a 1" × 10" × 10" board on top of two stacked tires. Make sure the tires are evenly stacked and centered.
4. A slide is easily constructed by placing a board on a climbing

structure. Make sure the board is properly finished. A few coats of Verathane will help in sliding.

Wooden spools that electric wire comes on are another possibility. Check with local electricians for their availability. Often you can get these free when you explain that you are a local day-care provider. You can use them in various sizes. A large spool can become a table, and small spools can be used for stools. The children will also enjoy climbing them.

Old packing crates can also be of value. These quickly become climbing structures, so make sure that they are sturdy.

Watch yard and rummage sales for riding toys or rocking horses. Inspect them before buying. Make sure they are sturdy enough for your day-care children, and they will add to the joy of outdoor play. The trick is to be on the watch for good finds. Someone else's castoff can become the major attraction in your outside play area. Look over each possibility carefully. Note needed repairs. Use your ingenuity to transform an old item into an exciting new one. Have fun creating your outside play area.

Whether you care for infants, toddlers, or preschoolers, ev- it often. Remember that, weather permitting, any activity that can be done inside can be done outside. You can read stories on the grass. Art projects can be done at a picnic table. Often these are less messy when done outside anyway.

Whether you care for infants, toddlers, or pre-schoolers, everyone will enjoy outside play. It can even be a welcome break for you. As the children play, you can sit and enjoy observing them. This can give you a new perpsective.

Teach your children how to use the outside play area properly. Although accidents will happen, there will be fewer if children follow a few basic rules:

1. Talk about courtesy. Explain how important it is to take turns.
2. Do not allow shoving, pushing, or chasing around or on play equipment.
3. Do not allow the play equipment to be overloaded with children.

4. Children should not have anything in their mouths (gum, candy, food) when playing on equipment.
5. Small toys, wagons, tricycles, should be kept away from outside play equipment.
6. Take time to demonstrate the proper use of each piece of play equipment to each child in your care.

Include your day-care children in planning safety rules. They will remember rules that they help make easier than ones you establish. Discuss all safety rules on a regular basis. Children need rules to be repeated to them so that they are not forgotten.

Remember that small children will need constant supervision. If children begin to tire out, take time for a short rest. This is a good time to share a snack. It will refuel their energy, rest their bodies, and maintain a sense of safety.

Be prepared for those occasional accidents. Have a first-aid kit available when playing outside. This will avert having to herd everybody inside to find a Band-Aid. It's a good idea to keep the first-aid kit handy at all times. Remember to wash any cut or scrape before applying a dressing.

Have fun in your outside play area with your day-care children. Together you can safely enjoy the outdoors and your day-care children can enjoy their creativity. With careful planning, you can look forward to saying yes to the question "Can we go outside now?"

Chapter 6

ACTIVITIES, GAMES, CRAFTS, BOOKS

"It's boring here! There's nothing to do." Rest assured that you are not the only provider who has ever heard this complaint. Children have short attention spans. When they lack a variety of new things to do, they loudly express their dissatisfaction. What then can you, as the provider, do to keep their days from becoming monotonous? The easiest solution is to do something fun together. When *you* take an active part, the children love it—which does make you feel *wanted*!

Activities, games, crafts, and books will provide you with endless ideas for entertaining projects to do together. Perhaps you could plan to include a weekly craft in your daily routine. Books read together offer the enjoyment of sharing quiet time, and games allow you to help the children to interact with each other socially. Activities can be as simple as a quiet walk, or as exciting as a field trip. Whatever you decide to do, the point is to enjoy doing it.

Children are always learning through the experiences they encounter on a daily basis. They need some quiet time, and they need time to be boisterous and active. The ideas that follow can be used daily, weekly, or monthly. You, as the provider, can choose anything that will fit into your schedule. Most ideas you'll find are very simple. Some have to be planned, others can be allowed to just happen.

THINGS TO DO TOGETHER

1. Tell stories with bag or finger puppets.
2. Describe pictures of all kinds.
3. Play dress-up.
4. Teach nursery rhymes.
5. Sing songs together.
6. Play recordings.
7. Have show and tell: each child brings something from home to talk about.
8. Watch *Sesame Street* or other quality program together and then talk about what you saw.
9. Talk to each child individually about favorite things (pet, name, color, story character).
10. Take a neighborhood walk and collect leaves, wildflowers (not neighbors' plantings!), or rocks.
11. Cut pictures out of magazines to make a collage.
12. Have children help make beds or set the table.
13. Play hopscotch together.
14. Draw and color, or paint, portraits. Let provider and children take turns as a model. Frame with cardboard. Decorate as desired.
15. Help children to roller-skate or jump rope.
16. Play ball together.
17. Name body parts and pieces of clothing: coat, hat, pants, shirt, hand, fingers, thumb, toes, head, arm, leg.
18. String beads, empty spools, popcorn, or Cheerios.
19. Draw shapes: circles, squares, stars, triangles, and talk about what comes in the shape drawn. Circle/sun; square/box.
20. Play guessing games: "Coffee Pot."
21. Visit your local firestation. Call first to set a time. Most firemen welcome young children if advance notice is given.
22. Bake cookies together.

THINGS TO DO TOGETHER (continued)

23. Test balance by walking the lines on the sidewalk; do broad-jumps.
24. On a hot day, give the children paintbrushes and pails of water to paint the sidewalk or the house. The water will evaporate, leaving nothing to clean up. Always supervise.
25. Visit a museum.
26. Start a small children's exercise class: play a favorite song while moving in a circle. March, sway, hop, swing arms, bend down, and bounce to the music.
27. Work a puzzle.
28. Play a game of Old Maid.
29. Play hide-and-seek; hide-the-thimble.
30. Teach as you shop: name products, colors, shapes.
31. Read a story.
32. Ride a city bus.
33. Visit an airport, train depot, or shipping dock
34. Put on a play: *Snow White, Cinderella, Robin Hood, Mary Had a Little Lamb, The Owl and the Pussy-Cat.*
35. Make a map of the house or neighborhood.
36. Count money: nickels, dimes, pennies, or quarters.
37. Climb a tree or jungle gym.
38. Swim at the neighborhood park.
39. Watch birds build nests.
40. Visit a farm, dairy, or zoo.
41. Plant seeds indoors or outdoors.
42. Sit outside and listen for sounds.
43. Have children make up stories about a picture you select.
44. Make your own puzzles by gluing magazine pictures on cardboard and then cutting into large pieces with scissors.
45. Have international days: children dress like children of another country. This can follow a simple study of geography or a story. Dressing in costumes fromother lands will help children to appreciate that all people are alike—only their dress, language, and customs are different.
46. Provide job bags: pillow slips filled with tools of the trade for hairdressers, carpenters, bakers, cowboys or girls, teachers, cobblers.

THINGS TO DO TOGETHER (continued)

47. Provide boxes or cartons to use as forts, playhouses, cars, or spaceships.
48. Play store.
49. Fly kites.
50. Make paper airplanes to fly.
51. Bake bread.
52. Make paper chains.
53. Have a parade, with banners, "floats," a "band," a "grandstand" for the "mayor."
54. Visit a local bakery.
55. Visit your local school for a music program.
56. Roast pumpkin seeds.
57. Classify a pile of bits and pieces as to size, shape, and color.
58. Hammer nails into old wood.
59. Start a sentence and let each child finish it.
60. Tour a fast-food restaurant: call in advance.
61. Play in a sandbox outside.
62. Use crayons to color in coloring books or freehand on paper. Frame each with construction paper to make it special.
63. Finger-paint on large sheets of butcher paper.
64. Build tents out of blankets.
65. Grow your own sprouts and shoots.
66. Feed the birds or the ducks.
67. Blow bubbles and chase them.
68. If it is hot, play with the hose outside. Supervise, so that children do not place their mouths over the nozzle.
69. Fish with magnets for paper fish with paper clips on their mouths.
70. Float boats in the sink.
71. Make a bird feeder.
72. Build cities out of blocks.
73. Encourage role-playing: mother, father, butcher, teacher, shopkeeper, mail carrier, plumber.
74. Play with a salt tray: fill a big roasting pan with a thick layer of salt. Let the children write, draw, swirl or become bulldozers. You can substitute oatmeal, cornmeal, rice, or dry cereal for indoors, sand for outdoors. Supervise closely.

THINGS TO DO TOGETHER (continued)

75. Color pictures and mail them to Grandma.
76. Let children play with an old typewriter.
77. Make rhythm shakers: fill tin boxes or cans with rice or beans.
78. Show the wonders of a magnifying glass.
79. Provide an old baby scale so that children can weigh their dolls.
80. Count cars, trees, flowers, dogs, or cats on a walk.
81. Take helium balloons, attach the child's name and address with a note to whoever finds the balloon to let the child know where it was found. Let them fly high.
82. Make bouquets of paper flowers for parents by glueing paper circles on paper stems and painting or coloring as desired.
83. Slide on cardboard down a grassy hill.
84. Go for a bike ride.
85. Allow children to run a vacuum, help with laundry, or dust the furniture.
86. Teach children to sew with a large needle, yarn, and pieces of fabric.
87. Take the children to a play or a movie.
88. Take photographs of each child, have them developed, and share them together.
89. Teach the children spatial concepts such as in and out, around and through, up and down.
90. Visit your public library.
91. If it's snowing: Build a snowman, go sledding, throw snowballs.
92. If it's raining: Bundle up and walk in the rain, watch gutters fill with water, look at the rain clouds, talk about where rain comes from and why.
93. Take paper flowers to a nursing home, neighbor, or friend.
94. Show children how telephones work.
95. Put on a magic show.

GAMES TO PLAY OR SING

1. Simon Says
2. Old Maid
3. Dominos
4. Checkers
5. Monopoly
6. The Ungame
7. Marble Games
8. Bingo
9. Hide-and-Seek
10. London Bridge
11. Ring Around a Rosy
12. Soccer
13. Baseball
14. Frisbee
15. Tic-Tac-Toe
16. Musical Chairs
17. Lotto
18. Slapjack
19. Follow the Leader
20. Mother, May I
21. Red Light, Green Light
22. Farmer in the Dell
23. Memory games
24. Hot Potato
25. There Once Was a Miller, and He Lived by the Mill
26. Loopy-Loo
27. The Wheels on the Car
28. This Old Man

The Touch Game

Put a few small items in a paper bag (doorknob, key, curler, Artgum, pinecone, stringbean). Have each child close her eyes, reach into the bag, and then tell you what is inside. For a variation, make this a sniffing game. Pass vanilla, soap, cinnamon, pencil shavings, pine needles under child's nose. Have him identify by the smell.

The Connecting Game

Put a rubber band, piece of cloth, piece of paper, Scotch tape, glue, bobby pin, safety pin, paper clips, feather, and a piece of string on a tray. Have the children look at each item and then find any two that can be connected together. Example: Scotch tape and paper or bobby pin and feather. The combinations are endless.

Find the Button

Hide a button or what-have-you. Give the children clues to find it. Let them know if they are getting warm or cold.

Draw a Man

Two or more children can participate. The object is to draw a man. Each child takes a turn drawing a different feature. For instance, one draws the head, another adds the body. Continue until the children are satisfied with the picture. For a variation: use long strip of paper from a roll of butcher wrap. Have children make a big picture that depicts "moving day," school, picnic at the park, or a circus. Each child adds his own interpretation.

Name Games

1. Name items that are easily associated with others. Such as: table/chair, salt/pepper, cup/saucer, pencil/paper. Begin by naming the item and allow the child to name the partner.
2. Name three items of the same color; have the child tell you the color. Let each one take turns. For instance, strawberries, cherries, and apples are red. You can vary this game by making it visual. Have the child find you three objects in your house that are red or any other color.

Clothespin in the Jar

Place a wide-mouth jar on the floor. Have children kneel on a chair and drop clothespins into the jar. Count how many each child gets or have them count each other's.

Classify Game

Using colored beads, different kinds of macaroni, or several kinds of dry beans, let the children put like kinds in cups. Or use animal cards to sort and classify as to farm animals, wild animals, animals that live in trees or holes, pets that live in cages, that go outside.

Matching Game

Allow children to match letters or numbers on blocks or cards. Also match feet with shoes, heads with hats, earrings with ears. You can even match clothing with the weather. For instance, say to the child: "If it is raining outside, what must I wear to play outside?"

Penny Game

Hide pennies around the house. Give the children specific directions to follow such as "Find the penny under the orange sofa." Allow the children to keep the pennies found.

Rattle Games for Baby

Rattles are fun for both baby and you. When both of you are in a happy mood, try a few of these games:

1. Lie baby on back, rotate rattle in circles about 12 inches above the face. Catch his eye so he can follow it.
2. Put baby on tummy, shake rattle and move it upward so that baby raises and lowers head. Talk lovingly to baby.
3. Play hide-and-seek with the rattle sound. Hide the rattle, shake it and let baby find it by the noise it makes. This will elicit squeals of triumph.

Balloon Game

Blow up enough balloons to give each child his own when the game is finished. Give the first child three balloons to toss, one at a time, into an empty laundry basket. Take turns to see how many each child can toss into basket.

"Telephone" Game

Have one child whisper a simple sentence to the next. Continue until each child has had a turn. The last child says aloud what he has heard. "I like you" can come out "Bite your shoe."

THINGS TO MAKE

Beanbags

You will need:

scissors
sand, rice, or dried beans
fabric scraps
needle and yarn

Cut fabric into desired shapes. To add dimension, cut sides, bottom, and top. Sew fabric together with needle and yarn, leaving an opening for filling. Fill with sand, rice, or dried beans and finish sewing.

Bird Feeder

You will need:

empty coffee can with plastic lid
aluminum pieplate
string
metal adhesive
can opener
birdseed

Make three openings in bottom and top side of can. Space these holes evenly. Attach string through holes in top to balance can for hanging. Glue bottom of can to center of inverted pie plate. Let dry. Fill with birdseed and place plastic lid on can. Hang in tree. Refill as necessary.

Bookmark

You will need:

colored paper
small magazine pictures
clear contact plastic
glue
scissors

Cut out a 2" x 5" piece of paper. Glue on small pictures. Cover with contact plastic and trim edges. Children could personalize theirs with drawings.

Boxes

Push-and-pull boxes are just boxes that are sturdy enough for babies to crawl into and children to push and pull.

Large boxes can be colored and designed by children to use as dollhouses or cars to ride in.

Robots can be made from boxes large enough to slip over heads. Cut holes for arms and decorate to make each robot an individual.

Finger puppets can be made from small lipstick boxes. Color in eyes, mouth, nose, hair, and clothes to make each puppet unique.

Villages can be made from small food boxes. Color each one to resemble a different building (gas station, bank, store, florist, school). Then assemble to lay out a village for small people.

Carrot Garden

Cut off about 2 inches of each carrot. Cut off any wilted leaves. Place cut carrots in a shallow bowl with cut ends down.

Place small pebbles around carrots to hold them down. Fill the bowl half full of water and place in a sunny area. New shoots will appear in about a week. Then plant the carrots in soil and watch them grow.

Collages

You will need:

construction paper
scissors
glue
magazine pictures
old greeting cards

Have the children cut out pictures with a theme (springtime, a picnic, the beach, traveling). Glue the pictures on a piece of construction paper. Make sure they cover the entire paper with pictures cut in different sizes.

Crystals in a Bowl

You will need:

a few rocks
a shallow bowl (glass)
6 tbsp. salt
6 tbsp. bluing
6 tbsp. water
1 tbsp. ammonia
food coloring

Place rocks in bottom of bowl. Combine salt, bluing, water, and ammonia in a small cup and mix well. Pour mixture over rocks. Add a few drops of food coloring over mixture. Allow to stand until crystals form. This usually takes a few hours and lasts a few days.

Cymbals

Tie ribbon bows on the handles of two pot covers. Make sure the pot covers are about the same size. Hit together!

Drum

Decorate an empty oatmeal box and lid. Attach a string to both sides to allow the drum to hang from the child's neck. To make drumsticks, place empty thread spools on the ends of unsharpened pencils.

Egg Cartons

1. To make bells, cover individual sections in foil. Attach a string to the top for hanging.
2. Clown's nose is simply one section painted red and threaded with elastic.
3. Multileg animal is one strip painted and decorated to resemble a caterpillar, centipede, or what-have-you.
4. A tower can be made by painting and then stacking several boxes on top of each other to reach desired height.
5. Storage containers can be made by decorating and filling. Use the cartons to hold jewelry, small toys, clips, pins.

Finger Puppets

You will need:

   construction paper
   yarn
   paper clip
   marking pens

Cut a piece of paper approximately 5 x 9 inches. Fold it in half and then half again lengthwise, leaving a long narrow strip. Curl the top half down and clip to the middle of the strip. Draw a face on the loop. Tie some yarn on the top for hair. You now have a finger puppet.

Finger Paint

You will need:

½ cup nonrising wheat flour
2 cups water
1 tbsp. glycerine
1 tsp. borax
food coloring
small jars with lids

Mix flour with ½ cup of water to form a paste. Put into sauce pan over low heat and add the remaining water. Cook until thick and clear, stirring constantly. Remove from heat and cool. Add glycerine and borax. Divide into small jars. Add desired food coloring to each jar and shake to disperse color. If mixture is too thick, thin with a few drops of water. Use shelf paper or typewriter paper to make pictures or designs. Keep paints sealed when not in use.

Leaf Rubbings

You will need:

white construction paper
crayons
tape
various leaves

Tape leaves to underside of paper. Have children rub color crayons over leaves on paper. The outline of the leaf will soon appear. Remove tape and leaf.

Lentil Forest

In a small saucer, spread a single layer of dry lentils. Add enough water to moisten, but do not allow the lentils to float.

Keep moist in a sunny area. In about 10 days the lentils will begin to sprout. Plant the lentils in soil and watch them grow.

Macaroni Necklaces

You will need:

yarn
macaroni (large shapes)
food coloring
sheet of wax paper

Divide macaroni into bowls. Add food coloring to each bowl. Gently stir macaroni to color evenly. Spread on wax paper to dry. When completely dry, thread yarn through holes in macaroni. Secure the ends to form necklace.

Magnets

You will need:

scissors
glue
small rocks
small plastic eyes
small cotton balls
6" strip of adhesive magnet

Cut magnet strip into six pieces. Take off paper covering adhesive and attach either a rock or a cottonball. Glue on plastic eyes. Keep on refrigerator doors to hang children's drawings.

Noisemaker

Remove the label from a clean plastic bottle. Partially fill with uncooked rice or dried beans. Fasten top. Decorate sides and attach a ribbon to the top. Shake to make a sound.

Paper Bag Masks

You will need:

- large paper bag for each child
- scissors
- colored paper
- glue
- crayons

Try bag on each child to find place for the eyes. Take bag off and measure eyes to make sure they are even. Cut out eyes. Use colored paper to cut out mouth, eyebrows, hair, ears. Allow children to personalize each mask with crayons. When completed, try on for hours of fun.

Paper Bag Tricks

Decorate lunch size paper bags to make hand puppets. Turn bags inside out to use for drawing or coloring. Make paper hats from paper bags. The paper is heavier and holds its shape longer.

Personalized Soap

You will need:

- bath size Ivory soap
- glue, canning wax
- favorite picture

Glue picture on soap bar. Allow to dry. Melt wax in an electric frying pan. Dip the soap, picture side down, into the hot wax. It will dry immediately.

Placemats

You will need:

- construction paper
- scissors

glue
crayons or markers
clear plastic Peel'n'Stick

Have children draw and color pictures on one sheet of construction paper. They can cut shapes out of a different color and glue them onto the paper for added dimension. Cover each one with plastic Peel'n'Stick on the front and the back. Trim edges in a scallop design.

Piñata

You will need:

large balloon
scissors
colored tissue paper strips
clothespin
powdered starch

Mix 3 cups of cold water and 1 cup of starch in a saucepan. Stir over low heat with wooden spoon until mixture becomes very sticky. Blow up balloon and secure tightly with string, leaving loop for hanging later. Rub starch mixture all over balloon. Dip tissue strips into starch and shake off excess. Carefully smooth each piece onto balloon, overlapping until balloon is covered. Hang with clothespin to dry overnight. When balloon is hard, puncture with pin to let out air. Decorate in brilliant colors. With scissors cut a small hole in top of balloon, add small pieces of candy, favors, or small lightweight toys. Hang for an exciting centerpiece.

Pinwheels

You will need:

2 4" x 8" pieces of paper
wooden stick

small nail
crayons

Color the paper in any design. Fold paper in half. Assemble two pieces of paper and wooden stick with small nail.

Potato Prints

You will need:

potato
sharp knife
paint
paper

Carve designs into the end of a potato. Dip into paint and make prints on paper or all-over pattern on old bedsheet, towel, or curtain.

Puppets

You will need:

old socks
felt pieces
fabric glue
scissors

Cut out eyes, nose, mouth, and ears from felt. Glue on old sock with fabric glue. Allow to dry. Put on a puppet show.

Paper Cup Puppet

You will need:

paper cup
yarn

glue
construction paper

Cut out a small circle on the front of the paper cup for the mouth. Draw eyes and nose or cut them out of construction paper and glue in place. Glue some yarn on top for hair. Stick a finger up under the cup and out of the mouth hole and make him talk.

Big Mouth Puppet

You will need:

paper plate
construction paper
cotton balls
glue

Fold a paper plate in half. Glue a strip of paper 2 x 4 inches on top for a finger holder. Glue on two cotton balls for eyes and two small dots of construction paper in the center of each. Cut out a long tongue and glue it inside the mouth. Slip your fingers through the top holder and put your thumb underneath to make the big mouth sing.

Walking Puppet

You will need:

light cardboard
markers
scissors

Draw a simple puppet figure on cardboard. Cut it out. Color on features with markers. Cut out two circles at the bottom of the puppet. Stick your fingers through the holes and make your puppet walk. You can vary this by cutting out any shape you wish (fruits, vegetables, tree, letters, or numbers).

Snoopy the Beagle

You will need:

- paper cups
- construction paper
- glue
- napkin
- scissors

Make a finger hole on the side of each paper cup. Cut out a 2-inch white circle, a ½-inch black circle, two circles for eyes, and two large oblong circles for ears. Glue the large white circle at the bottom of the side without the finger hole. Glue the small black circle on the large white one. This is the nose. Cut and glue a mouth below the nose. Glue on eyes and ears. Place on finger to make your puppet come alive.

Variation: Make large ears and a trunk to create an elephant or whiskers for a cat. Any animal can be made with a little imagination.

Snowman

You will need:

- cotton balls
- paper plates
- glue
- buttons
- yarn
- cinnamon sticks
- pencil

Draw a snowman in center of paper plate. Apply glue. Fill in with cotton balls. Glue buttons on for eyes and cinnamon sticks for arms. Allow child to decorate with buttons and yarn.

ACTIVITIES, GAMES, CRAFTS, BOOKS

Silver Box

You will need:

small box with lid
glue
crushed eggshells
silver paint

Decorate top and sides of box with glue and crushed eggshells. Allow to dry completely. Paint with silver paint and dry.

Snowflakes

You will need:

white typewriter paper
scissors
glue
black construction paper

Fold typing paper into quarters. Cut into all four sides, being careful not to cut the paper all the way across. The more holes that are made, the lacier the design will be. Mount the snowflake on the black construction paper.

Salt and Flour Clay

You will need:

1 cup salt
½ cup flour
1 cup water
food coloring

Combine salt and flour in a pan and add water. Heat over a very low flame, stirring constantly until mixture is thick and rubbery. Spoon onto a cookie sheet to cool. If it is too sticky after it has cooled, roll into a little flour. Store in an airtight container.

Wooden Musical Blocks

Use two pieces of wood approximately 4" long. An old 2 x 4 will do, if cut to desired length. Paint or color each piece. Slap blocks together in a back and forth motion.

BOOKS TO READ

Barrie, Sir James M. *Peter Pan.*
Baum, Lyman F. *The Wizard of Oz.*
Branco, Margery. *The Velveteen Rabbit.*
Bond, Michael. *Paddington at the Circus.*
Brown, Margaret Wise. *Goodnight Moon.*
Bruna, Dick. *Miffy at the Zoo.*
Bushnell, Catherine. *Raggedy Ann and Andy in the Tunnel of Lost Toys.*
Cleary, Beverly. *Ramona and Her Father.*
Craig, Bobbie. *A Comic and Curious Collection of Animals, Birds and other Creatures.*
DeRegniers, Beatrice. *Little Sister and the Month Brothers.*
Dwight, Revena. *Bert's Hall of Great Inventions.*
Disney, Walt. *Cinderella.*
Disney, Walt. *The Haunted House.*
Disney, Walt. *1,001 Dalmatians.*
Flack, Marjorie. *Angus and the Ducks.*
Funai, Mamori. *Make and Poki in the Rain Forest.*
Gackenbach, Dick. *Mother Rabbit's Son Tom.*
Gannett, Ruth Stiles. *My Father's Dragon.*
Garelick, May. *Where Does the Butterfly Go When It Rains.*
Graham, Kennon. *Land of the Lost.*
Harrison, David L. *The Book of Great Stories.*

ACTIVITIES, GAMES, CRAFTS, BOOKS

Haviland, Virginia. *Favorite Fairy Tales Told in France.*
Hazen, Barbara Shook. *Raggedy Ann and Andy and the Rainy-Day Circus.*
Hoff, Syd. *Stanley.*
Hoff, Syd. *Danny and the Dinosaur.*
Hurd, Edith Thacker. *Come and Have Fun.*
Joyce, Irma. *Never Talk to Strangers.*
Mayer, Mercer. *Little Monster's Mother Goose.*
McGovern, Ann. *Zoo, Where Are You.*
Milne, A. A. *When We Were Very Young.*
Milne, A. A. *Now We Are Six.*
Milne, A. A. *Winnie-the-Pooh.*
Milne, A. A. *The House at Pooh Corner.*
Payne, Emmy. *Kate-No-Pocket.*
Parrish, Peggy. *Dinosaur Time.*
Peck, Robert Newton. *Soup.*
Potter, Beatrix. *The Tale of the Flopsy Bunnies.*
Potter, Beatrix. *The Tale of the Squirrel Nutkin.*
Rey, Hans A. *Curious George.*
Rockwell, Anne. *The Three Bears and Fifteen Other Stories.*
Rounds, Glan. *Mr. Yowder and the Steamboat.*
Segal, Lore Groszmann. *Tell Me a Mitzi.*
Sendak, Maurice. *Where the Wild Things Are.*
Seuss, Dr. *One Fish, Two Fish, Red Fish, Blue Fish.*
Seuss, Dr. *And to Think That I Saw it on Mulberry Street.*
Stiles, Norman. *The Count's Number Parade.*
Stiles, Norman. *Farmer Grover.*
Thayer, Jane. *Gus and the Baby Ghost.*
Viorst, Judith. *Alexander and the Terrible, Horrible, No Good, Very Bad Day.*
White, E. B. *Charlotte's Web.*
Wiersum, Gale. *The Runaway Squash.*
Yolen, Jane. *No Bath Tonight.*

Chapter 7

CHILD-SAFE

As a day-care provider you have accepted an enormous responsibility in caring for young children. This responsibility must be first of all reflected in the safety precautions you take to make your home child-safe. Both parents and children trust you to provide an environment that is as safe as possible.

You will be alone with the children in your care for most of the day. You not only need to child-safe your home, but you must also plan for emergencies such as fire, accidents, and illness.

IN THE HOME

If, as the old saying goes, "A man's home is his castle," in a day-care home, "A child's special place is his haven." How can you make your day-care children's special place a haven?

Perhaps it is a good idea to first sit on the floor of each room, and get a feel of the room at the child's level and, as much as possible, from his point of view. Slowly look around the room for hidden dangers. Are the electrical outlets covered with plastic protectors? Are electrical cords to lamps, clocks, air conditioners, stereo, out of the sight of curious children? Are valuable vases, pictures, curios, put where a small child cannot accidentally break them? Remember, young children are very curious. They will open any drawer or cupboard. Think of this as you scan each room in your home.

Children's safety needs change as each child grows. Infants will roll off beds or sofas. Never leave them alone on a bed or sofa. If you must leave, spread a blanket on the floor, and then lay the infant on the blanket. The same is true for changing tables and cribs with the sides down. It only takes a second for an infant to roll and fall to the floor. Even a bassinet can be rocked over by a fussing baby.

When caring for infants, try to keep all diapering supplies in a convenient place. This will not only save you steps but you won't have to leave little Angie alone until one is found. Make sure all safety pins are kept out of reach. Even baby powder can be a hazard to infants if they inhale or ingest it.

Infant seats and high chairs are prized equipment in the day-care home, but they must be used with caution. Use infant seats only on the floor, or when you are carrying them. Babies' movements can tip the seats easily. Make sure that you fasten the safety belt when you put an infant in the seat. If left unfastened, the infant can easily squirm out the bottom. When using high chairs, fasten the safety belt too. Check the tray to make sure it fastens securely to the high chair. Many infants have been injured when they have pushed on the tray causing it to release, allowing the baby to fall to the floor.

Playpens must be used safely, too. Install a bumper pad inside to make sure that the baby will not hit his head on anything hard. Do not leave the side down. Babies can pinch their fingers when they move the unlatched side back and forth. Check the latches or locks to make sure they are in proper working order. Nursery equipment manufactured before 1974 may not conform to safety regulations. Take time to check all equipment carefully before using it. Make sure the mattress is firm and of proper size. Infants are constantly moving their small bodies, and can easily wedge their heads between the crib, or playpen side, and a loose mattress. This can, and has, resulted in suffocation. It is wise not to leave an infant unattended in either a crib or a playpen.

Remember that infants are helpless in water. They can easily drown in a very small amount. Never leave a baby alone in, or near, water for even a moment. When you bathe an infant, hold the head securely. Bath water should be tested with the elbow, not the hand. It should be at body temperature.

Infants will put anything in their grasp into their mouths. As you scan each room for hazards, be particularly aware of any object that may be swallowed. Put these objects out of the babies' reach.

Toddlers will seek out stairways, electrical outlets, closets, drawers, sinks, and tubs. Cleaning products, aftershaves, mouthwash, and anything else they may find may be drunk quickly. Lock all such items away from investigating babies. Install gates at stairways. Make sure all doors leading outside are locked to prevent these little people from wandering outside.

Anything that dangles from a table will be enthusiastically pulled down. Tablecloths, doilies, and plants should not be draped over the sides of tables.

Toddlers will climb on chairs, stools, tables, cupboards, drawers, desks, and bookshelves. Never let a small child see you put something they want on top of the refrigerator or a high cabinet. They will undoubtedly scale the obstacle when you are out of the room.

When cooking, keep all pot handles toward the back of the stove. This will help to avoid dangerous spillage. If possible, cook only on the back burners. Little ones are often tempted to peek at what you are preparing. If you are using the front burners, they may burn their fingers. Teach them that a stove is hot, and not to be played with. Use caution when opening oven doors. It only takes a moment for a toddler to touch a hot oven rack.

If you think that the hazards are overemphasized, just follow an active toddler around a room for a few minutes. Then multiply his exploits by the number of toddlers you will be caring for. The possible dangers will obviously increase with each additional toddler in your care. Two lively, curious toddlers can devastate a room within a few minutes.

Then, there are the two- and three-year-olds to protect. They are as curious as the toddlers, but they are not as cautious. They will open and shut all doors. Simple locks are easily undone. Their love of climbing knows no bounds. Windows are of special interest to them.

This makes it necessary to have all windows screened. If you have a two-story house, pay special attention to second-floor windows. Make sure the screens are secure. Many small children have fallen from windows that were improperly screened. No precaution is better worth the time it takes to check each window in your day-care home.

At this age, children are highly adventurous, and will wander off quickly. You must watch them carefully when they are outside. They can easily scale small fences if they want to, or unlatch gates.

Children who are two or three years of age often fail to watch where they are going. They run into walls, doors, swings, and each other. They will hit their heads on tables and counters. Even toys left on the floor will become a hazard.

Two-year-olds especially seem to trip over their own feet. This does not mean that you have to protect them from themselves. On the contrary, they develop coordination and self-confidence in the process of falling and getting back up. Children must be allowed to climb, jump, walk, crawl, and touch things to learn. But as a provider, you must make it safe for them to do such things.

Four- and five-year-olds seem mature when compared with two- or three-year-olds. They should have already learned the dangers of matches, open fires, stoves, and sharp objects. That does not mean that you can trust them completely around such items, though. Put matches, knives, and scissors away.

Children of this age are very independent. Often you will hear "I can do it by myself." Try not to discourage their independence. Instead, explain how to use an implement safely; let them know what has to be done under supervision. Four- or five-year-olds will listen to reason, if it is explained clearly.

You need to realize that this age group is very busy. They quickly move from one thing to another. Talking becomes their number one pastime, so they don't always watch where they are going when they are conversing. Streets are fascinating to them. It is important to teach them not only the dangers of streets, but also how to cross them properly. You will have to stress the importance of looking both ways continually.

They love to imitate mommy, daddy, and you. This often leads to quiet games of playing house. It can also lead to other things, such as trying to cook, answering the telephone, and even answering the door.

This may be the time to help your four- and five-year-old day-care children with personal safety. You can also include the younger children. Discuss "stranger-danger" with them. Stranger-danger is the awareness of who a stranger is, and why the children should be cautious. Remember, though, that to a small child any person whom they see more than once is not a stranger. For instance, the man who mows your neighbor's lawn may not be a stranger to them even if he is to you. Help them to understand the dangers of accepting rides in cars, or candy from someone without first asking you or their parents.

Ask your local police for information you could share with your day-care children. They usually give out such information through safety programs in elementary schools.

Teach your day-care children their full names, addresses, parents' names, your name, and telephone number. Even a two-year-old can memorize his full name and telephone number. Don't forget to teach them their area code. That way, if the unthinkable happens and they are lost or kidnapped, they will be able to call home.

It may take you extra time, but it is important to help your day-care children learn personal safety. After all, as their provider, you are with them the greater part of their waking hours. You become one of the most influential adults in their lives while they are in your care. The safety habits you instill in them now will be carried with them throughout their entire lives.

Children learn through example. If you are careful with scissors, knives, and appliances, they will follow your example. Every child is a unique, one-of-a-kind, and precious individual. So is every day-care provider. Practice safety together in your day-care home and be prepared for any and all emergencies.

SAFETY AND SANITARY PRECAUTIONS

In order for your home to be child-safe, you must be able to identify possible safety hazards in order to correct them. Check the following:

1. If you have a septic tank that shows any sign of seepage, have it serviced immediately.
2. Does your hot water heater have a safety release valve? Make sure it does. Also check the water temperature. Too hot water will scald. 110°–120° is suggested.
3. Insects and rodents carry disease. Eliminate any infestation before caring for children. Remember to store insect sprays out of children's access. Rodent traps must be where children cannot reach them.
4. If you live in an area where drainage ditches are found, do not allow children to play around them. Not only is drowning a possibility, but disease.
5. Inspect your yard on a regular basis. Remove any glass, nails, cans, and sharp sticks.
6. Use a garbage can with a lid that can be fastened inside your home. Empty all wastebaskets and kitchen garbage daily. Children often play in open garbage cans, and this can be dangerous.
7. Keep an emergency flashlight with batteries and a transistor radio handy. If the electricity goes off suddenly, you will be prepared to see and hear what's going on.
8. Keep diaper pails out of the children's reach, and fasten lids securely.
9. During electrical or severe wind storms, keep the children inside. In an electrical storm shut off the TV and the CB if you have one. Antennas may be hit by lightning. During a severe wind storm, stay away from windows, and draw the drapes to catch flying glass if the windows should break.
10. Keep children away from woodpiles.
11. Check fences on a regular basis for possible hazards. If you have chain link and the sharp barbs are up at the top, bend the barbs down with pliers.

12. Keep all sharp tools and electrical equipment locked away from children.
13. Make sure all bookcases are stable. Children often try to climb them.

FIRE PROTECTION

No one word can strike more terror in your heart than "fire." The word itself, when screamed, requires immediate action on the part of all who hear it. The home environment is particularly dangerous. According to the Fire Bureau, four out of five deaths due to fire occur in the home. In addition, many people suffer nonfatal burns each year. Prevention of burns is essentially a matter of preventing fires and of knowing escape routes in case of a home fire.

As a day-care provider, you have the responsibility for many children on a day-to-day basis. It is therefore essential to review the basic points of specific fire prevention.

1. Install fire extinguishers in kitchens, basements, garages, laundry rooms, and by fireplaces or wood stoves. Make sure they are accessible.
2. Know how to use a fire extinguisher. Visit your local fire station on a field trip with your day-care children. Ask the fireman to demonstrate how one works. Call ahead of time so they will be ready for children.
3. Repair or replace defective or inadequate electrical wiring.
4. Use only nonflammable cleaning fluids.
5. Hang clothes away from stoves or fireplaces.
6. Store flammable materials in a safe place.
7. Supervise children by any open fire.
8. Store matches and lighters out of children's reach.
9. Turn pot and pan handles to the back of the stove.
10. Install home fire detectors on each floor of your home.

More pointers could be included, but it is impossible to list every fire hazard. The main factor is to be aware of fire hazards, to eliminate as many of them as possible, and to have a plan of escape if a fire breaks out.

Every day-care home should have an established fire escape plan. Every child in your care should know what to do in case of fire. How do you make an escape plan? First, draw a layout of your house; include every room, doorway, and window. Second, identify two exits for each room (for example, one door and one window). Third, choose a meeting spot outside where everyone can meet after leaving the house. That way you can count heads. Fourth, discuss the plan with your day-care children. The two most important things to remember in case of a fire are to get everyone out of the house, and then to call the fire department.

Perhaps you can set aside a particular day each week or month to have a fire drill. In case of fire your day-care children need to react quickly. They cannot stop to pick up anything. Children will do whatever they have been trained to do in an emergency. Since it is easy to become confused in a crisis, children need to know exactly what they are to do if an emergency should occur.

In a fire, gases form quickly, and temperatures rise rapidly. Because heat and gas rise, the hottest temperatures and the most gas will be in the highest places. Therefore, smoke alarms should be installed on ceilings. This also makes it important for you to teach the children how to make a safe, fast exit out of habit. Stress the need to get help. That way, if you are unconscious, the children will know how to get assistance. Teach them how to call for help on the telephone. Some cities now have an emergency number to call such as "911." Tell the child to answer all of the questions that are asked. This is why, when teaching personal safety, it is important to teach your day-care children your own full name and address as well as theirs.

Fire departments are extremely concerned at overcrowding in day-care homes. They assume that the more children in care, the greater the risk of not being able to get everyone out of the home if a fire should occur. If you must care for an increased number of children, make sure that each child knows how to react in an emergency. You could even call the fire department to alert them that you are a day-care provider.

AUTO SAFETY

Occasionally you may have to drop off and pick up children at school, or you may take your group on field trips. Whatever the reason for driving, safety is the most important part of your journey.

Many states now have laws governing the use of seatbelts for children and adults. Even if your state does not require that children be buckled in a safety restraint, you should consider the consequences if they are not.

Some people feel that a small child can be protected in an auto accident by being held by an adult. Recent safety studies show this not to be the case. A small child weighing 30 pounds, when thrown in a 30-mile per hour impact, exerts a force of 1,000 pounds. How many pounds of force would you then exert against the dash with an infant in your arms? Obviously, it is safer for the infant and the small child to be buckled in.

The American Medical Association has recommended that a child over five years old, and weighing more than 50 pounds, should wear a seatbelt. A child under five years of age, and weighing less than 50 pounds, should be placed in specially designed, safety approved car seats.

Not every day-care provider is financially capable of providing three or four special car seats. You can ask the children's parents to leave their car seats, or you can check with local auto clubs where you might purchase some at reduced cost. Some organizations even rent car seats for a minimal fee. Purchasing your own may be the best choice. After all, most day-care providers care for children under five years old; so you should get a lot of use out of them. The expense is also tax-deductible.

Auto safety is just as important as home and fire safety. It is your obligation to protect the children in your care under all circumstances, in the home or on the road.

POISON PREVENTION

All parents worry about the possibility of their children being poisoned. This concern is greatly increased for day-care providers. How can you prevent a child from being poisoned? What precautions are needed regarding storage, use, and disposal of medicines, cleaning supplies, art supplies, and even mouthwash and aftershaves?

Think about the distribution of such supplies in your day-care home. How are hazardous substances stored? Are they away from foodstuffs? Do you store all products in their original containers, and are they clearly marked as to contents and antidote? Have you stored all poisonous substances out of the reach of children? Preferably, they should be in a locked cabinet or closet.

You must also follow the guidelines supplied for safe use of all drugs and chemicals. Be sure to read the labels and follow the directions exactly. If it is a liquid medication, shake it well before you use it. This will prevent you from administering a concentrated dose.

The presence of children makes it necessary for you to take extra precautions with the use of medications. Never leave chewable vitamins where children can get to them. Instruct your day-care children not to eat or drink anything without your permission. Use *Mr. Yuk* stickers on all poisonous substances. Children readily identify *Mr. Yuk* as something to avoid.

When disposing of poisonous substances, flush them down the toilet. Rinse the container, and then throw it away. Make sure all medicine and drug supplies are dated when purchased.

Learn what to do in case of accidental poisoning. Always keep activated charcoal (to bind poison), and syrup of ipecac (to induce vomiting) in your medicine cabinet. Know the phone number of the poison control center. Take first-aid classes to prepare you to handle emergencies. The Red Cross offers such classes at a minimal charge. All of these steps are necessary to help prevent accidental poisoning.

ILLNESSES

Every day-care home should be prepared to deal with emergency situations. These can include accidents, serious injuries, falls, concussions, convulsions, and sudden illnesses. Many day-care homes care for children with mild illnesses such as allergies, asthma, and the sniffles. As a provider, you must decide what constitutes an ill child in your home day-care. But, remember, you are not a medical authority. Do not make any medical diagnosis. Let the attending physician do that.

At one time or another, though, you will probably care for ill children. You should have some basic knowledge about childhood illnesses and methods of care. This information can be gathered by attending workshops, discussions, and demonstrations held by local physicians and county health nurses. Many areas now have health fairs that provide much information to the public free of charge.

You should have a medical history for each child in your care. Parents should provide this at the time of registration. They must update your information after medical examinations. Do not administer any medication to a child in your care without the parent's written authorization. Have them personally write the type of medication, the amount of the dose, and the times it is to be administered to the child. Make sure that the parents sign the permission for medication form.

When a child is ill, his needs should be uppermost in your mind. These include closer supervision, a restful environment, and several quiet activities. A small child needs extra attention when he is ill. If there is any change in his condition for the worse, notify his parents at once.

Some children may become suddenly ill because of a health hazard. You must be aware of possible hazards in order to help identify the reason for the sudden illness. Each changing season brings new health hazards to guard against. This is especially true of winter and summer.

Winter's cold weather causes problems as minor as chapped lips and as major as frostbite. Make sure that the children in your care are adequately dressed for the cold weather when playing outside. Keep some form of lip balm handy. Avoid overexposure by limiting the time spent outdoors. If children experience pain or numbness in their fingers or toes, seek medical advice immediately.

In the summer you have to be conscious of the possible hazards of the sun, the heat, the water, and also of food. To avoid sun hazards, follow these simple guidelines:

1. Between the hours of 11 a.m. and 2 p.m., when the sun is extremely hot, limit the childrens' outside play to a few minutes at a time.
2. Apply a sunscreen to the childrens' skin. Don't forget their noses. Reapply after swimming.
3. Keep hats on infants and toddlers to prevent their small heads from getting sunburned.
4. Do not allow children to take naps in the sun on a blanket. Even if it appears not to be very warm, sunburn is possible. Remember to make sure playpens are in the shade when outside.

To avoid heat hazards:

1. Avoid strenuous activity at midday.
2. Wear clothing that allows air to circulate through it.
3. Eat more frequent meals throughout the day, and eat less at each.
4. Know the symptoms of heat stroke and heat exhaustion. Learn first aid procedures for these illnesses.
5. Keep small bodies from dehydrating. Encourage children to drink lots of fluids. Water and fruit juices are especially beneficial. Avoid juices that have no nutritional value.

To avoid water hazards:

1. Never allow children to swim or wade unsupervised.
2. Avoid swimming immediately after eting, when overheated, or when physically tired.
3. If possible, teach all young children water safety. If you have a pool, teach young children water survival techniques. Contact your local "Y" for information on available classses. Water survival can even be taught to babies. Then, if they should accidentally fall into the pool, they will automatically float on their back, or hold onto the side until help arrives.
4. Do not allow a small child to put a running hose into his mouth. The force of the water could cause the child to choke, or even drown.
5. Use slip-and-slide devices with extreme caution. Do not allow the children to push or shove.

6. Never leave infants, toddlers, or small children alone in a wading pool.
7. Have children wear sandals when playing in lawn sprinklers. This will prevent them from being stung by bees that have been attracted by the water.
8. Children should always wear safety-approved flotation devices when in pools.

To avoid food hazards:

1. Wash your hands thoroughly before preparing food. Wash after touching raw meat, poultry, or eggs.
2. Avoid using foods containing milk, cream, or eggs on picnics.
3. Keep cold foods chilled properly at 40 degrees in portable ice chests.

A word of caution:

If you are not sure that a particular activity is completely child-safe, substitute another until you have had a chance to think all of the "kinks" out of it. Keeping your day-care children safe is the main reason that you are such an important person— to those children, their families, and the community.